T714

New Approaches to Cancer Treatment
Unsaturated Lipids and Photodynamic Therapy

New Approaches to Cancer Treatment

Unsaturated Lipids and Photodynamic Therapy

Edited by

David F. Horrobin MA DPhil BM BCh
Scotia Research Institute, Kentville,
Nova Scotia, Canada

CHURCHILL LIVINGSTONE
EDINBURGH LONDON MADRID MELBOURNE NEW YORK AND TOKYO 1994

CHURCHILL LIVINGSTONE
Medical Division of Longman Group Limited

Distributed in the United States of America by Churchill
Livingstone Inc., 650 Avenue of the Americas, New York, N.Y.
10011, and by associated companies, branches and
representatives throughout the world.

First published 1994

ISBN 0443 050821

British Library Cataloguing in Publication Data
A catalogue record for this book is available from the British
Library

Library of Congress Cataloging in Publication Data
A catalogue record for this book is available from the Library of
Congress

Typeset by Saxon Graphics Ltd, Derby
Printed in Great Britain by Biddles Ltd, Guildford, Surrey

Contents

SECTION 2
Photodynamic therapy

Contributors

Allan L. Abramson
Department of Otolaryngology and Communicative Disorders, Long Island Jewish Medical Center, The Long Island Campus for the Albert Einstein College of Medicine, New Hyde Park, New York, USA

Hans-Jorg Altermatt
Department of Pathology, University of Bern, Bern, Switzerland

Ulrich Althaus
Department of Thoracic and Cardiovascular Surgery, University of Bern, Bern, Switzerland

Raymond Bonnett
Department of Chemistry, Queen Mary and Westfield College, London, UK

David C. Carter
Department of Surgery, Royal Infirmary, Edinburgh, UK

J. Stuart Falconer
Department of Surgery, Royal Infirmary, Edinburgh, UK

Kenneth C. H. Fearon
Department of Surgery, Royal Infirmary, Edinburgh, UK

John W. Hopewell
CRC Normal Tissue Radiobiology Research Group, Research Institute (University of Oxford), Churchill Hospital, Oxford, UK

David F. Horrobin
Scotia Research Institute, Kentville, Nova Scotia, Canada

John O. Hunter
Gastroenterology Research Unit, Addenbrooke's Hospital, Cambridge, UK

W. G. Jiang
Department of Surgery, University of Wales College of Medicine, Heath Park, Cardiff, UK

A. Lee
Gastroenterology Research Unit, Addenbrooke's Hospital, Cambridge, UK

Chung K. Lim
Medical Research Council Laboratories, Surrey, UK

Lennart A. Lofgren
Department of Otolaryngology and Communicative Disorders, Long Island Jewish Medical Center, The Long Island Campus for the Albert Einstein College of Medicine, New Hyde Park, New York, USA

Gerard M. Morris
CRC Normal Tissue Radiobiology Research Group, Research Institute (University of Oxford), Churchill Hospital, Oxford, UK

Bernhard Nachbur
Department of Thoracic and Cardiovascular Surgery, University of Bern, Bern, Switzerland

May Nouri
Department of Otolaryngology and Communicative Disorders, Long Island Jewish Medical Center, The Long Island Campus for the Albert Einstein College of Medicine, New Hyde Park, New York, USA

Malcolm C. A. Puntis
Department of Surgery, University of Wales College of Medicine, Heath Park, Cardiff, UK

P. Dominic Reynolds
Gastroenterology Research Unit, Addenbrooke's Hospital, Cambridge, UK

Mohi Rezvani
CRC Normal Tissue Radiobiology Research Group, Research Instititute (University of Oxford), Churchill Hospital, Oxford, UK

Hans-Beat Ris
Department of Thoracic and Cardiovascular Surgery, University of Bern, Bern, Switzerland

Michael E. C. Robbins
CRC Normal Tissue Radiobiology Research Group, Research Institute (University of Oxford), Churchill Hospital, Oxford, UK

Avigdor M. Ronn
Department of Otolaryngology and Communicative Disorders, Long Island Jewish Medical Center, The Long Island Campus for the Albert Einstein College of Medicine, New Hyde Park, New York, USA

Graham A. Ross
CRC Normal Tissue Radiobiology Research Group, Research Institute (University of Oxford), Churchill Hospital, Oxford, UK

Mark J. Shikowitz
Department of Otolaryngology and Communicative Disorders, Long Island Jewish Medical Center, The Long Island Campus for the Albert Einstein College of Medicine, New Hyde Park, New York, USA

Willem Star
Dr Daniel den Hoed Cancer Centre, Rotterdam, The Netherlands

Betty M. Steinberg
Department of Otolaryngology and Communicative Disorders, Long Island Jewish Medical Center, The Long Island Campus for the Albert Einstein College of Medicine, New Hyde Park, New York, USA

J. Charles M. Stewart
Scotia Pharmaceuticals Ltd, Guildford, Surrey, UK

Michael J. Tisdale
CRC Nutritional Biochemistry Research Group, Pharmaceutical Sciences Institute, Aston University, Birmingham, UK

Quita Tuffnell
Gastroenterology Research Unit, Addenbrooke's Hospital, Cambridge, UK

Gerard J. M. J. van den Aardweg
CRC Normal Tissue Radiobiology Research Group, Research Institute (University of Oxford), Churchill Hospital, Oxford, UK

Nynke van der Veen
Dr Daniel den Hoed Cancer Centre, Rotterdam, The Netherlands

Eric van Leengoed
Dr Daniel den Hoed Cancer Centre, Rotterdam, The Netherlands

Quian Wang
Medical Research Council Laboratories, Surrey, UK

Elizabeth M. Whitehouse
CRC Normal Tissue Radiobiology Research Group, Research Institute (University of Oxford), Churchill Hospital, Oxford, UK

Unsaturated lipids

1. Unsaturated lipids and cancer

D. F. Horrobin

INTRODUCTION

There are many anti-cancer drugs which are cytotoxic in vitro and capable of shrinking cancers in vivo. There are, however, many problems associated with their use. The most important is their toxicity to normal tissues. Other major problems are:

1. Many cancers are resistant to cytotoxic drugs.
2. Even cancers which are initially sensitive often become resistant.
3. Ability of a drug to shrink a tumour is often rather poorly correlated with prolongation of life.

If a drug has little effect in prolonging life and at the same time produces serious toxicity, many patients and their doctors may feel that shrinkage of the cancer size has relatively little meaning.

The mechanisms of action of most cytotoxics are not yet fully certain but there is increasing evidence that for many of them the ability to generate free radicals in target cells is fundamental. Free radicals contain an unpaired electron and are able to react destructively with nucleic acids and with unsaturated lipids. The latter reaction results in a cascade of substances, often called by the somewhat catch-all phrase 'lipid peroxides'. The particular importance of the reactions with unsaturated lipids is that they are self-regenerating chain reactions in which more and more free radicals are formed (Fig. 1.1). These chain reactions can be broken only by the activities of the chain-breaking anti-oxidants such as the tocopherols[1,2].

Anti-cancer agents capable of generating free radicals and lipid peroxides include ionizing radiation[1,3], *cis*-platin[4,5] doxorubicin[6-8], and bleomycin[9]. In patients treated in vivo with combination chemotherapy regimens including such agents as the vinca alkaloids, doxorubicin, cyclophosphamides, *cis*-platin and 5-fluorouracil free radical production in polymorphonuclear leucocytes has been shown to be enhanced[10].

Most attention has been paid to the interactions between free radicals and nucleic acids. However, it may well be that the free radicals interact with nucleic acids in part through the mediation of products of lipid peroxidation. It is not always appreciated that the nuclear material contains

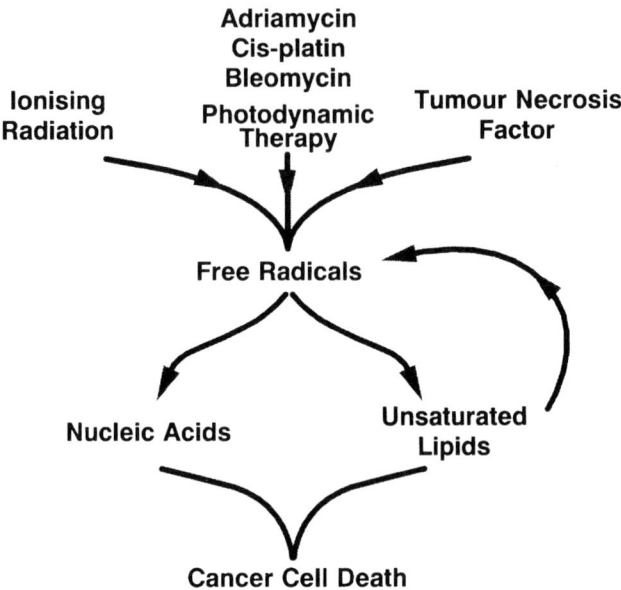

Fig. 1.1.   An outline of the relationship between various anti-cancer agents and the generation of free radicals and lipid peroxidation.

lipids which appear capable of interacting closely with DNA[11-13]. That the lipids probably have functional roles in this respect is indicated by the fact that the unsaturated lipids such as linoleic acid[14], and their derivatives, prostaglandin E_1 for example[15,16], are able to protect nucleic acids against the clastogenic actions of radiation and chemicals[15,16].

If free radical formation and lipid peroxidation are important in destroying cancer cells, then the aim of ideal cancer therapy would be to find an agent which would have these effects in cancer cells but not in normal tissue (Fig. 1.2). If this aim could be achieved one would have an anti-cancer agent akin to Ehrlich's magic bullet, a drug which could destroy one set of living cells, occupying territory in a living organism without damaging the normal cells of that organism. To date, this aim has been pursued primarily through the concept of selective targeting. Drugs are used which are toxic to both normal and malignant cells but by various techniques such as monoclonal antibodies to malignant cells, or selective uptake by the LDL-receptor route which is expressed more in malignant cells than in normal tissue, the toxic drugs are located primarily in the cancer cells. The approach described in this chapter is different. The drugs reach both malignant cells and normal cells to an equal extent. But because of fundamental differences in lipid metabolism between normal and malignant tissues, the drugs kill the cancer cells while leaving the normal cells unharmed.

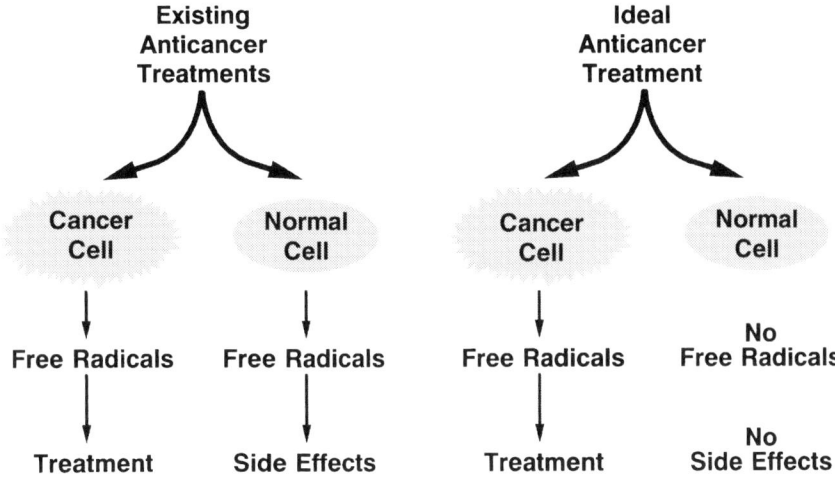

Fig. 1.2.   The ideal anti-cancer agent would selectively harm cancer cells without harming normal cells.

BACKGROUND

Unsaturated fatty acids

In saturated fatty acids the carbon atoms in the backbone of the fatty acid are linked by single bonds. In unsaturated fatty acids one or more of the carbon–carbon links is a double bond. By convention, fatty acids containing two or more double bonds are known as polyunsaturated.

The most important polyunsaturated fatty acids (PUFAs) in the body are the essential fatty acids (EFAs). There are two families of these, derived from linoleic acid (n-6 series) and alpha-linolenic acid (n-3 series) respectively (Fig. 1.3). The EFAs are termed essential because none of them can be manufactured de novo by mammals and so they must be taken in the diet[17-19]. The parent fatty acids, linoleic and alpha-linolenic, can however be converted within the body by a series of alternating desaturation reactions in which hydrogens are removed and new double bonds are formed, and elongation reactions in which two carbon atoms are added to the chain. There are five commonly identified metabolites of both linoleic and alpha-linolenic acids. Each of these metabolites probably has a specific role in the body, particularly important metabolites being dihomogammalinolenic acid (DGLA) and arachidonic acid (AA) of the n-6 series, and eicosapentaenoic acid (EPA) and docosahexaenoic acid (DHA) of the n-3 series.

The EFAs have many roles within the body[17-21]. They are required for the normal structure of all membranes including cell membranes, mitochondrial

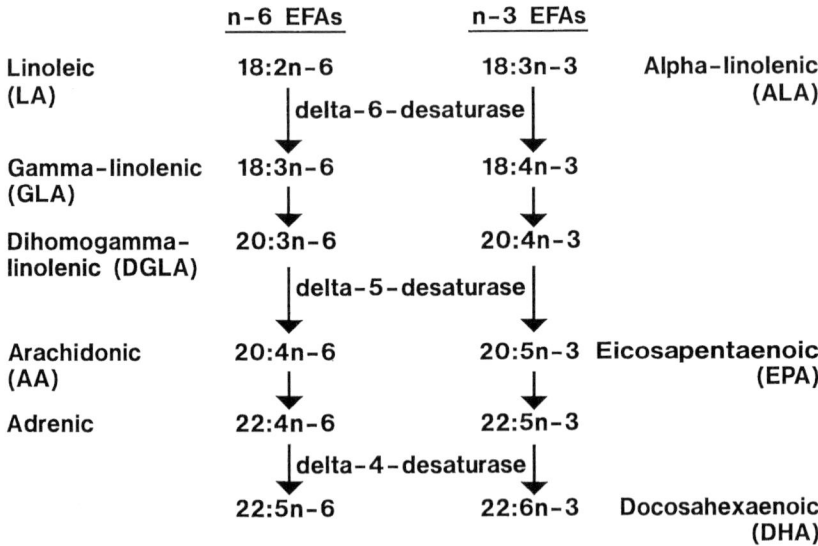

Fig. 1.3.   An outline of the metabolic pathways of the essential fatty acids.

membranes and nuclear membranes. They are precursors of a whole series of second messengers, including prostaglandins, leukotrienes and other molecules into which oxygen has been introduced and which are generally known as the eicosanoids. They are required for the normal transport of cholesterol around the body[17]. Very recently it has been recognized that the unsaturated fatty acids have a whole range of other effects including interaction with almost all second messenger systems and regulation of the formation of cytokines, and modulation of the behaviour of most membrane-bound proteins including receptors, ion channels and ATPases[22].

The EFAs are not the only biochemically important unsaturated fatty acids. In the EFAs, the double bonds are always separated by two carbon atoms in a methylene configuration, a configuration which is known as unconjugated. In conjugated double bonds there is no methylene carbon configuration between adjacent double bonds. Conjugated fatty acids are very highly susceptible to peroxidation. They are not usually found in substantial amounts in natural products or in the mammalian organism but they are readily formed from the EFAs during oxidative processes such as cooking[23]. There are some natural sources of conjugated unsaturated fatty acids such as the seeds of plants like *Impatiens balsamina* which contains substantial amounts of parinaric acid[24].

Peroxidation in cancer cells

All intact cells contain large amounts of highly unsaturated lipids. These lipids ought to be very susceptible to oxidation with the consequent production of a cascade of lipid peroxides.

Yet this does not happen. Lipid peroxides are found in normal cells, but at relatively low concentrations, and there is no explosive destruction of unsaturated lipids. This is partly because the lipids are compartmentalized and protected from oxygen and partly because there are effective systems both for preventing oxidation and for removing oxidized lipids which may be formed. Vitamin E is particularly important in preventing lipid peroxidation in the lipid phase and it interacts with vitamin C which is the key aqueous phase antioxidant. Systems involving glutathione and selenium are important both in resisting oxidation and in removing any peroxidized lipids which may be formed.

When cells are homogenized, the structural relationships which are important in resisting lipid peroxidation are destroyed and the process can occur rapidly. It can be monitored in a variety of ways, none of which is fully satisfactory. Common techniques involve the measurement of the formation of conjugated dienes from linoleic acid, or of the production of superoxide radicals, or of the production of malondialdehyde, an end-stage product of the lipid peroxidation process, or of electron paramagnetic resonance. All have their drawbacks and it is important not to overinterpret results obtained by one method. Transition metals such as iron and copper are powerful pro-oxidants and they are often added to reaction mixtures to enhance the rate of lipid peroxidation.

The most important single observation made on cancer cells in relation to lipid peroxidation is that such cells are unusually resistant. They always form much lower levels of lipid peroxides than do normal cells from the same tissue. This is an old observation, possibly first made by Donnan in the late 1940s[25], confirmed in the late 1950s[26,27] and repeated with the same results by many investigators since[28-38].

The loss of lipid peroxides is not an all-or-nothing phenomenon but bears a quantitative relationship to the degree of malignancy of the cancer. If hepatomas are divided into those which are growing slowly and those which are growing quickly, then the fast ones have the lowest rates of peroxidation, while the slower ones have intermediate peroxidation rates[31]. Moreover, the loss of peroxidation is not a late event in the development of malignancy but is a very early one. On exposure of tissues to carcinogens, even preneoplastic foci which occur before the development of frank malignancy can be shown to have reduced rates of peroxidation[34,38].

Lipid peroxidation as a normal regulator of cell division

There have been repeated suggestions that oxidation of lipids, far from being simply a pathological process, may be one of the key regulators of cell division. If this is so it implies that lipid peroxidation must be under strict metabolic control.

The first clue pointing in this direction was the observation that cells entering mitosis sharply reduce their consumption of oxygen and effectively become anaerobic[39,40]. Then it was observed that rapidly dividing normal cells, like cancer, have relatively low levels of lipid peroxidation[41-47]. Most convincingly, in rats which are partially hepatectomized and which are entrained to a strict light/dark and feeding cycle, the waves of cell division in the regenerating liver occur in coordinated waves with rest periods in between[29,42,43]. Immediately before and during cell division, the rate of lipid peroxidation is sharply reduced but rises rapidly again as the wave of division comes to an end and enters the quiescent phase. This influence of lipid peroxidation on cell division in normal tissues is a subject which deserves much more intensive investigation.

Mechanism of reduced lipid peroxidation in malignancy

There are three fundamental reasons why cancer cells might be unable to generate lipid peroxides normally. These are that they might contain excessive amounts of antioxidants, that they might contain inadequate amounts of highly unsaturated lipids to act as substrates, or that they might have particularly effective systems for eliminating free radicals and lipid peroxides[44].

The last of these possibilities can be eliminated because it is clear that cancer cells, given the right conditions, are capable of generating large quantities of lipid peroxides[45] and also that they have a reduced ability to remove superoxide radicals which may be involved in the process of lipid peroxidation[46,49].

There is substantial evidence for both of the first two possibilities. Initially most attention was paid to the concept that malignant cells may contain excessive amounts of antioxidants. There is no doubt that cancer cells are unusually rich in antioxidants and particularly in vitamin E[29,32,34]. In women with breast cancer, contrary to what might have been expected, vitamin E levels were higher than normal[48]. It has been suggested that one of the reasons why cancers often seem to grow more rapidly in children and young adults is that antioxidant activity is higher in young people than in older ones[34].

As well as being rich in vitamin E, malignant cells are also often rich in oleic acid[49,50,51]. It is not always appreciated that, for reasons which are not fully understood, oleic acid is an extremely effective antioxidant and is found in high concentrations in rapidly dividing tissues[52].

However, evidence is now accumulating to the effect that the most important factor in the reduced lipid peroxidation of malignant cells is the reduced availability of substrates in the form of highly unsaturated fatty acids. Cancer cells have low levels of unsaturated lipids with three or more double bonds as compared to normal cells[27,29,30,49,50,53,54]. The reduction in unsaturated fatty acids is greater, and the faster growing is the tumour[49]. The degree of depletion of unsaturated fatty acids in a malignant cell line in vitro can be an accurate predictor of its malignancy in vivo. If a range of mouse fibroblast mutants derived from a single parent cell line are arranged in order of malignancy, then the most malignant have lipids which are least saturated[55-57].

The reason for the reduced levels of highly unsaturated fatty acids in many malignant tissues is not yet certain. The observed changes could be caused by reduced formation of these fatty acids from the parent linoleic and alpha-linolenic acids or an increased rate of destruction or both. If there is an increased rate of destruction, normal EFA metabolism may be unable to compensate. This is because the first step in EFA metabolism, delta-6-desaturation (Fig. 1.3)[20,21] is slow and rate limiting. Fatty acids beyond that step which are rapidly lost may not be able to be replaced normally.

There is substantial evidence that in many malignant cells there is an impaired ability to form the highly unsaturated metabolites from dietary precursors. Transformed and malignant cell lines very frequently show loss of delta-6-desaturase or greatly reduced activity of the enzyme[58,59]. In a range of liver cancers of different types and of different origins, there is undoubtedly loss of the ability to convert linoleic acid to its metabolites[60-65,72]. Human lung cancer, transplanted into nude mice, has lost any ability to desaturate linoleic acid[66]. On the other hand, other malignant cell lines do exhibit some 6-desaturase activity, especially for alpha-linolenic acid and so the enzyme is certainly not always lost in malignant tissue[67-71]. It is therefore possible that both inadequate formation of highly unsaturated fatty acids and increased destruction by as-yet undefined mechanisms both contribute to the low levels found in cancer tissue.

Unsaturated lipids and metastasis

As has already been mentioned, cell lines show an inverse relationship between malignancy on implantation and the unsaturated fatty acids level of the membrane[55-57]. There are similar relationships between unsaturated lipid levels and the metastatic potential of cell lines.

Highly metastatic B16–F10 melanoma cells had lower levels of arachidonic acid and other unsaturated lipids than did the less metastatic B16–F1 cells[73]. However, Calerini et al found low levels of highly unsaturated fatty acids and high levels of oleic acid in both cell lines with no major difference between the two in fatty acid composition[74]. On the other hand, highly metastatic B77-AA6 3T3 fibroblasts showed lowered levels of arachidonic acid docosahexaenoic acid than did the less metastatic B77 cells[75]. Highly metastatic DU-145 human prostate cancer cells had much lower arachidonic acid levels than the less metastatic ND-1 cells.[75] More complex results were obtained with another pair of prostate cancer cell lines, with some polyunsaturates being higher and others lower in the more metastatic cells[76]. It is therefore apparent that more work needs to be done in this area. It should be noted that in human breast cancers in vivo, a high level of polyunsaturated fatty acid in the cancer predicted a low risk of future metastasis: low levels of EFAs in contrast predicted a high rate of metastasis[77] (Fig. 1.4). Evidence from the behaviour of human cancers in a clinical situation must certainly outweigh that from in vitro studies.

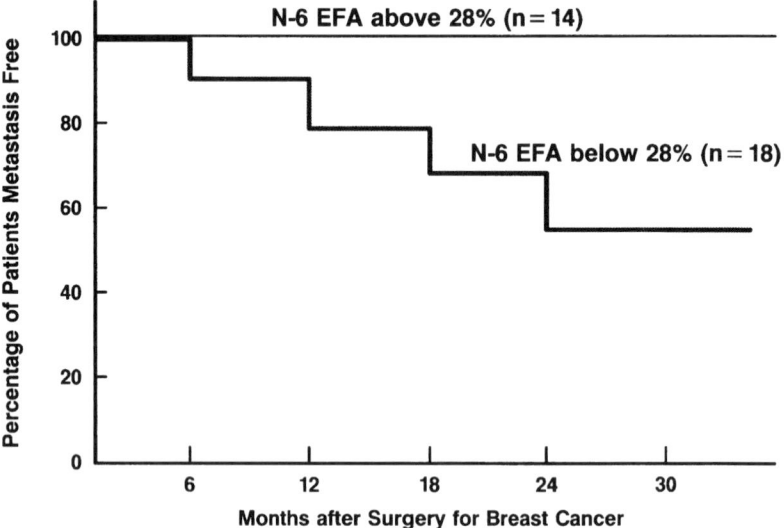

Fig. 1.4.   Occurrence of metastases following surgery in breast cancer in relation to the concentrations in tumour phosphatidyl-ethanolamine of n-6 essential fatty acids. (Data from reference 77.)

UNSATURATED LIPID EFFECTS ON MALIGNANT CELLS

The question of the importance of the reduced levels of unsaturated lipids found in malignant tissues can only be resolved by testing the effects of adding these lipids to cancers. This can be done with regard to cancer cell lines in vitro, to animal models of cancer in vivo, and ultimately to human cancers in patients.

Effects in vitro

Although there was much evidence by 1980 concerning deficits of unsaturated lipids in cancer cells, for some reason the simple experiment of testing the effects of addition of these lipids had never been performed. This is probably because the major emphasis of the research was related to the idea that the reduced lipid peroxidation characteristic of malignancy was primarily related to excess accumulation of antioxidants.

When fatty acids were tested on malignant cells for the first time, the rationale was different. In the 1970s a number of investigators had shown that artificially transformed cells could be made to behave normally by the addition of cyclic AMP to the culture medium or by the stimulation of endogenous cyclic AMP synthesis by prostaglandin (PG) E_1. Because of its instability, PGE_1 has serious limitations as a therapeutic agent, and so I proposed that a stable precursor of PGE_1 such as DGLA or gamma-linolenic acid (GLA) might be used instead[78]. It was felt that linoleic acid would be inappropriate because of evidence that malignant cells might be unable to convert linoleic acid to GLA normally[58,59].

The proposed hypothesis, namely that GLA and DGLA might be able to control cancer by inducing 'reverse transformation', was first tested by several groups of investigators in South Africa. They reported that GLA did not induce reverse transformation but was actually able to kill a range of malignant cells, including ones from liver, bone, breast, oesophagus and stomach[79-84]. The key observation was that cell death usually did not occur until after 5–7 d of incubation. The effect was therefore not a short-term cytotoxic one. The effects were also reported from my own laboratory and have now been repeatedly confirmed elsewhere. To my knowledge over 30 human cancer cell lines have now been tested in the presence of GLA and related essential fatty acids.[44,79-115] These cell lines now include all the common cancers including breast, lung, prostate, melanoma, liver, oral cavity, oesophagus, stomach, pancreas, uterus, colon, bone and leukaemias. In contrast, no normal cell lines have been harmed by concentrations of fatty acids which are able to kill malignant cells. These effects of the fatty acids in selectively killing cancer cells are similar to the effects of water soluble auto-oxidation products of unsaturated fatty acids.[86] They are also similar to some effects of unsaturated lipids on malignant cells which were reported in the early 1960s[87]. The results are consistent across all cancers and the key points which can be concluded from the many published papers[45,79-115] are summarized below:

1. Fatty acids with two or more double bonds are consistently able to kill malignant cells in culture whereas oleic acid, with one double bond, either has no effect or stimulates cell growth. When a range of different fatty acids is tested in the same system, the fatty acids with 3, 4 or 5 double bonds, especially GLA, DGLA, arachidonic acid and EPA, are consistently the most effective[45,85,88]. Linoleic acid with two double bonds and, surprisingly, docosahexaenoic acid (DHA) with six double bonds are relatively ineffective.

2. GLA and DGLA have no harmful effects on normal cells at the con-

centrations which kill malignant cells. EPA is also relatively harmless to normal cells but does exhibit some cytotoxic effects. AA also harms malignant cells much more than normal cells but exhibits cytotoxic effects on a substantial number of normal cells[44,45,88].

3. While some cytotoxic effects may be detectable in some cell lines by the third day, cell death rarely occurs before the fourth day following exposure and may not take place until the eighth or ninth day.

4. The effect is dose dependent. There are a few very sensitive cell lines, but most require a concentration of over 1×10^{-5} mol/l to have an effect. Almost all cell lines are killed at concentrations of 2×10^{-4} mol/l although a few may require higher concentrations.

5. The effects cannot be explained by gross differences of lipid uptake between normal and malignant cells. Indeed the malignant cells tend to take up rather less unsaturated fatty acid than normal cells[116]. However, in the malignant cells there is accumulation of lipid in droplets which can readily be observed microscopically, a phenomenon which occurs to a much smaller degree in normal cells.

6. When normal fibroblasts and human cancer cells are co-cultured, the cancer cells usually completely overgrow and destroy the normal cells. If an appropriate level of GLA is added to the culture, exactly the reverse takes place, with the normal cells outgrowing the malignant cells, and the latter dying[60].

Mechanism of cell killing

While much of the detail remains to be elucidated, there can be no doubt that the killing of the cancer cells involves the generation of free radicals and lipid peroxides. These substances are formed to a much greater extent in the cancer cells than in the normal cells. This rules out the hypothesis that low levels of lipid peroxides in cancer cells are attributable to an inability of cancer cells to make these compounds and suggests instead that cancer cells may actually produce excessive amounts if exposed to appropriate conditions. It also suggests that unsaturated fatty acids may indeed be true magic bullets, agents which reach both normal and malignant cells but which generate lethal amounts of cytotoxic free radicals and lipid peroxides only in the malignant cells leaving the normal cells unharmed (Fig. 1.2). There are many papers which all indicate that increased lipid oxidation and free radical generation is the basis of cell killing:

1. On exposure to GLA or other appropriate lipids, cancer cells generate large amounts of the end product of lipid peroxidation, malondialdehyde (MDA)[44,45,88,93,95,98,99,102,106,107,113,114]. Conjugated diene formation and production of peroxyl groups also correlate with cell death[109-111]. Some specific metabolites formed from GLA in malignant cells but not in

normal cells have now been identified[117]. Superoxide formation appears to be important in several cell lines[56,101,102,115] but not in all[113]. When normal cells are transformed by oncogenes or other means, they become much more sensitive to the cytotoxic effects of the polyunsaturated fatty acids and at the same time generate more lipid oxidation products[118,119].

2. The importance of lipid peroxidation is indicated by the fact that iron and copper consistently enhance both the cytotoxic effects of unsaturated fats and their ability to form lipid peroxides[44,45,88,109,110,111] whereas antioxidants such as vitamin E consistently inhibit both cytotoxicity and peroxidation. Hydroxyl radicals and hydrogen peroxide may not be involved since mannitol, a hydroxyl scavenger, and catalase, which destroys hydrogen peroxide, do not interfere with cytotoxicity[44]. Selenium and glutathione peroxidase which reduce peroxide levels, and superoxide dismutase which reduces superoxide, all attenuate the cytotoxic effects[44].

3. Products of the cyclo-oxygenase and lipoxygenase enzyme systems seem to have little role in the cytotoxicity. Inhibitors of these enzymes rarely interfere in any way with the cytotoxic effects[44,45,88,92,97,99].

Effects on metastatic potential

To date, most of the work has been done on the cell-killing effect in vitro. Relatively little has been done on the effects of fatty acids on the ability of cell lines to metastasize following short duration or sub-lethal exposure to the fatty acids. However, the colony-forming ability (which may reflect metastatic potential) of a series of rat brain cancer cell lines was markedly reduced following incubation of cells with GLA or EPA[119]. This is similar to the reduced tumour-forming potential of fibroblast lines incubated with polyunsaturated fatty acids[55-57]. Further, murine melanoma and human fibrosarcoma cell lines have been shown to exhibit reduced invasiveness, reduced production of collagenase, and reduced ability to produce lung metastases following exposure in vitro to EPA[120].

Modulation of conventional drug cytotoxic effects

Existing cytotoxic drugs are ineffective against many cancer cell lines. Moreover, cancers which once were sensitive to cytotoxics may become insensitive, not only to one drug but to many (the phenomenon of multi-drug resistance (MDR)). It is therefore not surprising that a good deal of effort has been put into investigating the possibility that unsaturated fatty acids may be able to modify the actions of existing anti-cancers. It is perhaps unfortunate that much of the work has been done using docosahexaenoic acid (DHA). Although this is the most highly unsaturated readily available fatty acid, it is now known that it is one of the less effective fatty acids as far as the actions against cancer cells are concerned. Much of the work would therefore bear repeating with the fatty acids with 3–5 double bonds.

Exposure of cell lines to DHA is able to enhance the sensitivity of cancer cells to both adriamycin and *cis*-platin[121–125]. The main effect seemed to be either on increased transport of the drug into cells or on reduced outward transport because the levels of the cytotoxic drugs inside cells increased[124,125]. Conjugates of 2-deoxy-5-fluorouridine (5d FU) with DHA were considerably more cytotoxic than 5d FU itself[126]. In this case, the actual conjugate seemed to be important since enhanced cytotoxicity was not observed when cells were simply incubated with both 5d FU and DHA.

GLA and DHA were both able to enhance the cytotoxicity of vincristine in vincristine-resistant neuroblastoma cells[127]. As with the other drugs, the fatty acids seemed to be able to increase the intracellular concentrations of vincristine.

Another way of enhancing the cytotoxic effect of adriamycin has been proposed with respect to liver cancer. This is to link the drug to arachidonic acid (AA). The rationale is that AA binds very strongly to alpha-fetoprotein, a protein which is produced in large amounts by liver cancer cells. The AA binding, it was thought, would help to localize the adriamycin in the cancer cells. Whatever the mechanism, an increased cytotoxic effect was indeed obtained[128].

Modulation of cytokine cytotoxic effects

A number of cytokines, notably interferons, tumour necrosis factor (TNF) and interleukin-2 have been proposed as possible drugs for use in cancer. In general, initial enthusiasm has led to the view that therapeutic effects are modest, toxicity is severe and that while there is indeed a place for these agents as anti-cancers their position is likely to be a limited one.

However, to date, one very important factor has been overlooked, This is that interferon[129–132], interleukin-2[133,134] and (TNF)[135,136] all require EFAs as components of the second messenger systems whereby they act on cells. If, as documented in this chapter, malignant cells tend to have low levels of the necessary EFAs, the effects of these cytokines on cancer cells might be very considerably enhanced by replenishing the EFA levels in these cancer cells. Moreover, this might enable desirable therapeutic effects to be achieved at much lower cytokine concentrations and so with many fewer side effects.

There are already a few studies which point in this direction but much more work is required to elucidate the full range of possibilities. Interferon requires EFAs to exert its antiviral actions[129–132], modulate phospholipid metabolism[137] and stimulate the production of free radicals[138]. It would therefore not be surprising if interferon effects on the cancers known to be susceptible to it were potentiated by the presence of EFAs.

With regard to TNF, a clone of a WEHI mouse fibrosarcoma has been identified which is highly susceptible to TNF in the presence of certain fatty acids but much less sensitive in their absence[139]. In particular, the parent EFAs, linoleic and alpha-linolenic acids, had little effect on the cytotoxicity of TNF.

In contrast, both n-3 and n-6 metabolites beyond the desaturation stage, including GLA, DGLA, AA, EPA and DHA, all considerably potentiated the cytotoxicity of TNF. This suggests that in cells in which 6-desaturation is slow or absent, TNF may have only modest cytotoxic effects but that these could be enhanced substantially by provision of the missing fatty acids.

Modulation of cachexia

There is good evidence that EPA and, to a lesser extent, GLA, may be able to inhibit cachexia due to malignancy. This is documented in detail in Chapter 2.

Modulation of thermal sensitivity

There is modest but increasing interest in the effect of hyperthermia as a treatment for cancer. There is good evidence that pre-exposing malignant cells to DHA is able to enhance their susceptibility to death by hyperthermia[12]. Arachidonic acid has a similar effect and it is possible that it may be working by enhancing thermally induced peroxidation[140].

ANIMAL STUDIES

Large numbers of studies have demonstrated that an increased intake of dietary linoleic acid is able to promote the development of various animal cancers, particularly of mammary cancer. It is possible that these studies may provide a case history as to how misleading animal experiments may be[44,141]. No epidemiological study in humans has ever shown that high intakes of linoleic acid are associated with breast cancer. If anything, the reverse is the case, especially when studies are conducted on cancers occurring within population groups. A large study of breast and other cancers in American nurses showed no significant association between linoleic acid and cancer[142]. The non-significant trend was in a direction opposite to that predicted from the animal studies, namely that the group with the lowest intake of linoleic acid showed the highest incidence of breast cancer. Women who later develop breast cancer had lower linoleic acid levels than matched controls[142a] while women whose cancers metastasized had lower tumour linoleic acid levels than those whose cancers did not[77]. Women with breast cancer have significantly lower levels of linoleic acid and arachidonic acid in red cells than did controls[142b]. In tissue from meningiomas[142c] and from prostatic cancers[142d] arachidonic acid levels were significantly lower than in corresponding non-cancerous tissue.

As yet there have been only limited animal studies on the effects of either n-3 or n-6 EFAs beyond the rate-limiting 6-desaturation step. Most of these studies have concerned the effects of diets supplemented with EPA and DHA in the form of fish oils. Fish oils have been reported to inhibit the growth of animal mammary and colon cancers[143-146]. They have also inhibited the growth in nude mice of human colon, lung, breast and melanoma cancers[147-149]. The effect seems to be related to lipid peroxidation since the inhibitory action of fish oil on breast cancer is enhanced by iron and inhibited by vitamin E[150].

A word of caution may be required, however, concerning the anti-cancer effects of high fish-oil doses. Fish meal enhanced the growth of a rat chemically induced colon cancer[151], increased pulmonary metastases of a Yoshida sarcoma in rats[152] and enhanced growth of the RDM4 lymphoma in mice[155], possibly by impairing lysis by LAK cells.

The experiments on fish oil which have shown inhibition of cancer growth as compared to the experiments with linoleic acid-rich vegetable oils which have consistently shown enhancement of animal cancer growth[153] have almost all been interpreted as indicating that n-6 EFAs enhance growth while n-3 EFAs inhibit it. This is almost certainly an incorrect observation. Comparing fish oil with linoleic acid is not only comparing n-3 EFAs with an n-6 EFA, it is also comparing n-3 EFAs with more than two double bonds and which are beyond the 6-desaturation step with an n-6 EFA which has only two double bonds and which is prior to the 6-desaturation step (Fig. 1.1). What happens when the correct experiments are done and fish oils are compared with n-6 EFAs beyond the point of 6-desaturation?

The answer is rather clear. All the work has been done using gamma-linolenic acid (GLA, 18:3n-6)-containing oils since other n-6 EFAs are not yet available for experimental purposes. Such GLA-containing oils are at least as effective as fish oils on a molar basis at inhibiting the growth of a variety of cancers. GLA-containing primrose oil was first shown by two separate groups to inhibit the growth of the R3230AC rat mammary cancer[154,155]. GLA-containing oils could also inhibit the growth of DMBA-induced mammary cancers in rats[143,156,157]. Two other groups have shown no effect of GLA-rich oils on a rat mammary cancer and a murine sarcoma[158,159] and a small stimulating effect on growth of a murine melanoma[160,161], an effect which was reversed, with inhibition of the tumour growth, when vitamin C was added to the diet[161]. The animal experiments most relevant to human cancers are ones in which human cancers are transplanted into nude mice. GLA-containing primrose oil had a striking inhibitory effect on both human breast cancer and human melanoma transplanted into nude mice, an effect which on a molar basis was considerably greater than that for EPA and DHA[162,163]. Both the ability of tumour cell injections to initiate cancers in nude mice, and the ability of those cancers which were initiated to then grow were inhibited[162,163] (Figs 1.5 and 1.6)

It should not be forgotten that even linoleic acid may inhibit the growth of cancers other than breast cancer. This effect has been shown for colon cancer[164] for a T cell lymphoma[165], for renal tract cancers[166], for an adrenal cortical cancer[167] and for a lymphoma[168]

The generalization that is commonly made in reviews, namely that n-3 EFAs inhibit cancer growth whereas n-6 EFAs promote it, is therefore quite inappropriate. Nearer the truth, but still too broad, is the idea that fatty acids of both n-6 and n-3 series which are beyond the 6-desaturation step are able to inhibit cancer growth.

HUMAN STUDIES

There seems little doubt that most and perhaps all human cancer cells in vitro can be killed by adequate concentrations of GLA, DGLA, AA and EPA. The concentrations required, particularly in the cases of GLA, DGLA and EPA, have few adverse effects on normal cells. Oral administration of very high doses of GLA and EPA has been shown to inhibit the growth of several animal cancers and of human cancers transplanted into nude mice. Can this laboratory work be transferred to human patients?

The animal studies have involved administration of the EFAs in the approximate range of 1–5% of total dietary calories. If we assume that a person is consuming 2500 kcal/d then this means 25–125 kcal as GLA or

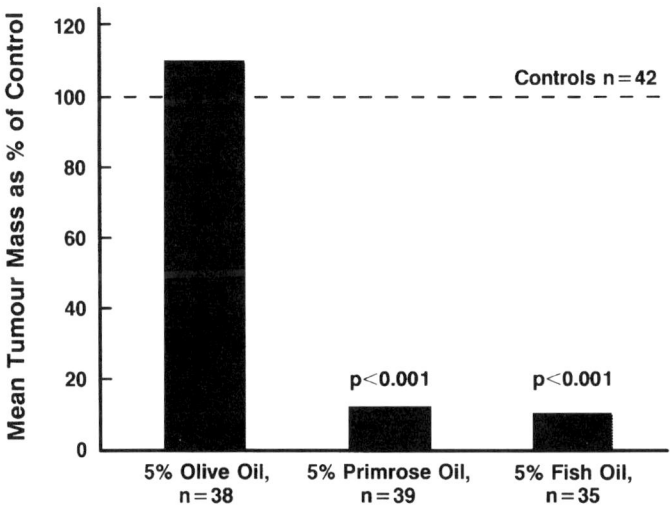

Fig. 1.5.   The growth of human melanoma cells transplanted into nude mice treated in four different ways: control, no addition to the diet: 5% olive oil in the diet: 5% primrose oil containing gamma-linolenic acid: 5% fish oil containing eicosapentaenoic acid. (Data from reference 162.)

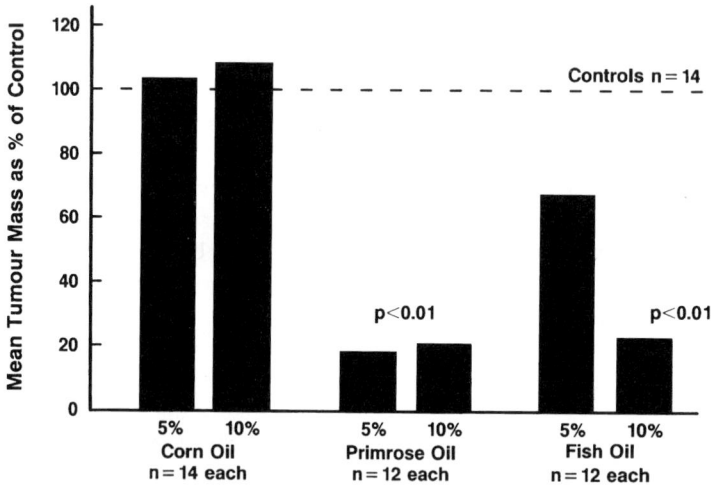

Fig. 1.6. The growth of human breast cancer cells transplanted into nude mic treated with various additions to the diet: control, no addition: 5% and 10% corn oil containing linoleic acid but no gamma-linolenic acid or eicosapentaenoic L: 5% and 10% primrose oil containing gamma-linolenic acid: 5% and 10% fish oil containing eicosapentaenoic acid. (Data from reference 162.)

EPA or in the region of 3–14 g of the pure acid. These amounts are difficult to tolerate orally because of gastrointestinal upsets. Moreover, when administered orally the fatty acids are likely to reach the blood in the forms of triglycerides, cholesterol esters and phospholipids. Not all tumours may have the metabolic machinery required to ensure delivery of the GLA or EPA from these lipid fractions to the cells in appropriate concentrations.

There have been two attempts to treat human cancers with oral GLA. A controlled study in colon cancer of 240 mg of GLA per day had no effect on survival[160]. However, this dose was almost certainly too small. Much higher doses of 700–1500 mg of GLA/d in the form of 9–18 g of evening primrose oil did appear to have beneficial effects in patients with liver, brain, lung, stomach and oesophageal cancers[170]. Two patients with mesothelioma appeared to respond well[170]. Although there were no important adverse effects other than gastrointestinal upsets consequent upon the large volumes of oil, the patients had considerable difficulty in taking the large numbers of capsules required.

Because of the difficulties with large amounts of oral lipid and because of the uncertain distribution of the fatty acids following this route of administration, it was decided to try to develop an intravenous formulation of GLA. A triglyceride emulsion was a possibility but was rejected because of the uncertain evenness of distribution in the extracellular fluid with this formulation. Free fatty acids are bound to albumin and released to all tissues via the medium of the plasma and extracellular fluid: as cells consume free fatty acids the equilibrium requires fatty acids bound to albumin to be released. It was therefore felt that this was likely to be the route which would ensure the most consistent distribution of the GLA throughout the body. The aim was to reach all the cancer cells, whether in the primary tumour or in metastases. In vitro cancer cells require exposure for 4–8 d before they die and so it was decided to administer the fatty acids intravenously for 10–15 d in order to mimic the in vitro conditions.

For ease of administration we wished to administer the GLA in aqueous intravenous fluids such as isotonic saline. The salts of the EFAs are relatively water soluble. If prepared in a concentrated solution of around 1 g of the salt in 10 ml of 20% ethanol, the material can readily be added to 500 ml of saline without precipitation. There were three salts to choose from, sodium, potassium or lithium. It was unwise to use potassium because of its cardiac effects. Lithium had the advantage over sodium of being useful in monitoring the rate of infusion. Fatty acids and their salts disrupt cell membranes, including those of red cells, by a detergent effect. In vitro studies showed that little haemolysis took place at concentrations below 10^{-3} molar, a concentration more than adequate to kill cancer cells on the basis of the in vitro evidence. Whereas fatty acid concentrations can be monitored only over hours and require specialized analytical techniques not routinely available in most hospitals, lithium concentrations can be monitored within minutes by flame photometry or on capilliary samples at the bed side using ion-selective electrodes. It was soon established that lithium-GLA monitoring was indeed a very useful, rapid technique for monitoring the lithium-GLA infusions and ensuring that substantial haemolysis did not occur.

A dose escalation study in patients with inoperable pancreatic cancer is described in Chapters 4, 5 and 6. Provided that central venous administration under appropriate heparin cover is used and provided that the dose is escalated slowly with monitoring of lithium levels, there seem to be no important adverse effects of lithium-GLA. The limiting toxicity is haemolysis produced by daily doses of between 5 and 20 g in most patients. Provided that the appropriate daily dose is not exceeded no limiting cumulative dose toxicity has been reached at doses up to 1.5 g/kg. It is possible that there may be no cumulative toxic limit provided that the daily limit is not exceeded. The toxicity of lithium is not a limiting factor. The target level of lithium is below 0.7 mmol/l, while a concentration of 0.8–1.0 mmol/l is used in many psychiatric clinics. Moreover in the treatment of cancer these lithium levels are maintained only for 1–3 weeks whereas in psychiatry higher lithium levels may be maintained for many years.

The initial dose escalation studies show a highly significant relationship between increasing dose of lithium-GLA and increasing survival. The highest doses of the drug are associated with an approximately four-fold increase in median survival, more than has been reported to date in response to any chemotherapy or radiotherapy regime in inoperable pancreatic cancer. A randomized, controlled phase III trial is now in progress, and the outcome of this must be awaited before anything definitive can be claimed about the effects of lithium-GLA on survival in pancreatic cancer.

The patients with pancreatic cancer prior to treatment showed severe deficits of the unsaturated fatty acids in red cell membranes (Fig. 1.7). This supports the view that these unsaturated lipids may be deficient in pancreatic cancer. After treatment with lithium-GLA the concentrations of the GLA metabolites, dihomogammalinolenic acid and arachidonic acid, rose significantly (Fig. 1.8).

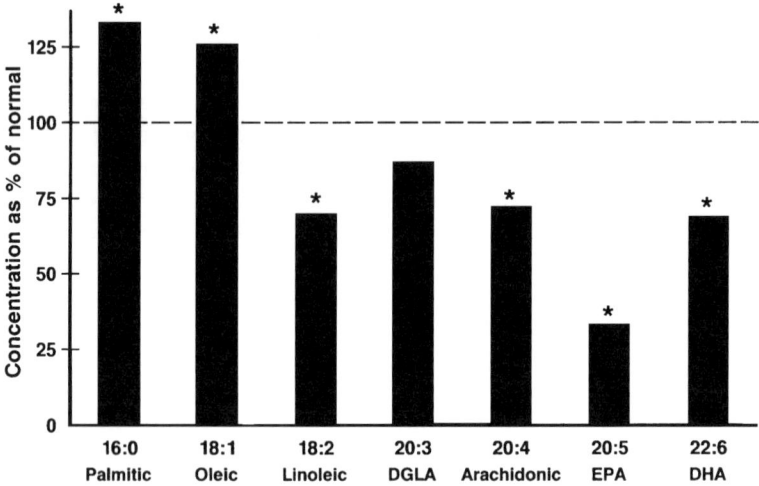

Fig. 1.7. The concentrations of the main fatty acids in the red cell membrane phospholipids of patients with pancreatic cancer. The concentrations of the unsaturated fatty acids are consistently lower than in normal control individuals. *Patients ($n = 24$) significantly different from controls ($n = 319$) at $P < 0.001$.

CONCLUSIONS

Polyunsaturated lipids with 3, 4 or 5 double bonds offer a promising new development in the management of human cancers without the generation of severe side effects. The results from cell culture and animal studies are consistent. Once the problems of delivering adequate concentrations of appropriate forms of the fatty acid to all cancer cells are solved, a proper evaluation of this new approach can take place. However, this delivery is simpler than in the case of most anticancer agents: the lack of harmful effects on normal cells means that the drugs can be delivered in adequate concentrations to all cells but only cancer cells will be harmed. The lithium salts of the fatty acids offer a promising delivery route which is currently being tested.

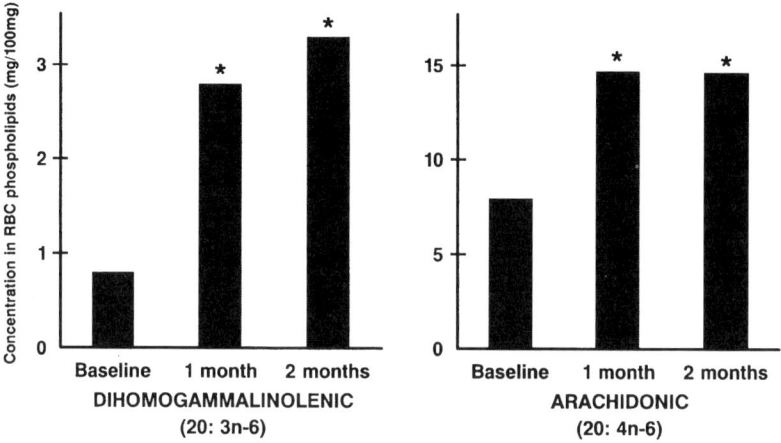

Fig. 1.8.   The changes in red cell phospholipids of patients with pancreatic cancer of the main metabolites of gamma-linolenic acid in response to infusions of lithium gammalinolenate. An infusion over 10 d produces a prolonged change in red cell membrane composition lasting at least 2 months. *Significantly different from baseline at $P < 0.01$.

REFERENCES

1.   Halliwell B, Gutteridge JMC 1985 Free radicals in biology and medicine. Oxford University Press, Oxford
2.   Dormandy TL 1983 An approach to free radicals. Lancet ii: 1010–1014.
3.   Barber AA, Wilbur KM 1954 The effect of X-radiation on the antioxidant activity of mammalian tissue. Radiation Research 10: 167–175.
4.   Sodhi A, Gupta P 1986 Increased release of hydrogen peroxide and superoxide anion by murine macrophages in vitro after *cis*-platin treatment. International Journal of Immunopharmacology 8: 709–714
5.   Sugihara K, Nanakano S, Koda, et al 1987 Stimulatory effect of cisplatin on production of lipid peroxidation in renal tissues. Japanese Journal of Pharmacology 43: 247–252
6.   Meijer C, Mulder NH, Timmer-Boscha H, et al 1987 Role of free radicals in an adriamycin-resistant human small cell lung cancer cell line. Cancer Research 47: 4613–4617
7.   Benchekroun MN, Robert J 1992 Measurement of doxorubicin-induced lipid peroxidation under the conditions that determine cytotoxicity in cultured tumour cells. Analytical Biochemistry 201 (2): 326–330
8.   Keizer HG, Pinedo HM, Schuurhuis GJ, Jeonje H 1990 Doxorubicin (adriamycin): a critical review of free radical-dependent mechanisms of cytotoxicity. Pharmacology and Therapeutics 47: 219–231
9.   Kanofsky JR 1986 Singlet oxygen production by bleomycin. Journal of Biological Chemistry 261: 13546–13550
10.   Sangeetha P, Das UN, Koratkar R, Suryaprabha P 1990 Increase in free radical generation and lipid peroxidation following chemotherapy in patients with cancer. Free Radical Biology & Medicine 8: 15–19
11.   Rose HG, Frenster JH 1965 Composition and metabolism of lipids within repressed and active chromatin of interphase lymphocytes. Biochimica et Biophysica Acta 106: 577–591
12.   Manzoli FA, Muchmore JH, Bonora B, et al 1974 Lipid-DNA Interactions. II. Phospholipids, cholesterol, glycerophosphorylcholine, sphingosine and fatty acids.

Biochimica et Biophysica Acta 340: 1–15

13.   Khan Z, Ariatti M, Hawtrey AO 1987 Studies on the interaction of DNA with neutral lipids and phospholipids. Medical Science Research 15: 1189

14.   Norman A, McBride WH, Bennett LR, et al 1988 Rapid communication. Postirradiation protection of chromosomes by linoleate. International Journal of Radiation Biology 54 (4): 521–524

15.   Das UN, Ramadevi G, Rao KP, Rao MS 1985 Prostaglandins and their precursors can modify genetic damage induced by gamma-radiation and benzo(a)pyrene. Prostaglandins 29: 911–919

16.   Sridevi K, Rao KP 1992 Anticlastogenic action of prostaglandin E, in human lymphocyte cultures. Medical Science Research 20: 677–678

17.   Sinclair HM 1990 History of essential fatty acids. In: Horrobin DF (ed) Omega-6 essential fatty acids: pathophysiology and roles in clinical medicine. Alan Liss, New York, pp 1–20

18.   Rivers JPW, Frankel TL 1981 Essential fatty acid deficiency. British Medical Bulletin 37: 59–64

19.   Holman RT 1988 George O Burr and the discovery of essential fatty acids. Journal of Nutrition 118: 535–540

20.   Horrobin DF 1990 Gamma-linolenic acid. Reviews of Contemporary Pharmacotherapy 1: 1–41

21.   Horrobin DF 1992 Nutritional and medical importance of gamma-linolenic acid. Progress in Lipid Research 31(2): 162–194

22.   Nunez EA 1993 Fatty acids and cell signalling. Prostaglandins Leukotrienes and EFAs 48: 1–122

23.   Pariza MM, Ha YL 1990 Conjugated dienoic derivatives of linoleic acid: mechanism of anticarcinogenic effect. Mutagens and carcinogens in the diet. Wiley-Liss, New York, pp 217–221.

24.   Cornelius AS, Yerram NR Kratz DA, Spector AA 1991 Cytotoxic effect of cis-parinaric acid in cultured malignant cells. Cancer Research 51: 6025–6030

25.   Donnan SK 1950 The thiobarbituric acid test applied to tissues from rats treated in various ways. Journal of Biological Chemistry 182: 415–419

26.   Shuster CW 1955 Effects of oxidised fatty acids on ascites tumour metabolism. Proceedings of the Society of Experimental Biology and Medicine 90: 423–427

27.   Ohnishi T 1952 Lipid peroxide formation and phospholipid in normal and tumour tissues. Gann 49: 233–248

28.   Burlakowa EB 1955 Bioantioxidants and synthetic inhibitors of radical processes. Russian Chemistry Review 44: 871–880

29.   Cheesman KH, Burton GW, Ingold KU, Slater TF 1984 Lipid peroxidation and lipid antioxidants in normal and cancer cells. Toxicology and Pathology 12 (3): 235–239

30.   Utsumi K, Yamamoto G, Inaba K 1965 Failure of ferrous iron induced lipid peroxidation and swelling in the mitochondria isolated from ascites tumour cells. Biochimica et Biophysica Acta 105: 368–371

31.   Bartoli GM, Galeotti T 1979 Growth related lipid peroxidation in tumours, microsomal membranes and mitochondria. Biochimica et Biophysica Acta 574: 41

32.   Lash ED 1966 The antioxidant and pre-oxidant activity in ascites tumours. Archives of Biochemistry and Biophysics 115: 332–336

33.   Neifakh EA, Hogan VE 1969 Accumulation of lipid peroxides in the organs of tumour-bearing animals in vivo. Biokhimiya 34: 692–698

34.   Duchesne J 1967 A unifying biochemical theory of cancer, senescence and maximal life span. Journal of Theoretical Biology 66: 137–145

35.   Galeotti T, Borrello S, Minotti G, et al 1984 Lipid composition, physical state and lipid peroxidation of tumour membranes. Toxicology and Pathology 12(4): 324–330

36.   Galeotti T, Borrello S, Palombini G, et al 1984 Lipid peroxidation and fluidity of plasma membranes from rat liver and Morris hepatoma 3924A. FEBS Letters 169(2): 169–173

37.   Cheeseman K, Emery S, Maddix S, et al 1988 Studies on lipid peroxidation in normal and tumour tissues. Biochemical Journal 250: 247–252

38.   Bendeti A 1984 Loss of lipid peroxidation as an histochemical marker for preneoplastic hepatocellular foci of rats. Cancer Research 5712–5717

39. Stern H, Kirk P 1948 The oxygen consumption of the microspores of *Trillium* in relation to the mitotic cycle. Journal of General Physiology 31: 243–248
40. Stern H 1956 Sulfhydryl groups and cell division. Science 124: 1292–1293
41. Cornwell DG, Morisaki N 1984 Fatty acid paradoxes in the control of cell proliferation: prostaglandins, lipid peroxides and oxidation reactions. In: Pryor WA (ed) Free radicals in biology. Academic Press, New York, pp 95–148
42. Wolfson N, Wilbur KM, Bernheim F 1956 Lipid peroxide formation in regenerating rat liver. Experimental Cell Research 10: 566–568
43. Cheeseman K, Collins M, Maddix S, et al 1986 Lipid peroxidation in regenerating rat liver. FEBS Letters 209: 191–196
44. Horrobin DF 1990 Essential fatty acids, lipid peroxidation and cancer. In: Horrobin DF (ed) Omega-6 essential fatty acids: pathophysiology and roles in clinical medicine. Alan R Liss, New York, 351–378
45. Begin ME, Ells G, Horrobin DF 1988 Polyunsaturated fatty acid-induced cytotoxicity against tumour cells and its relationship to lipid peroxidation. Journal of the National Cancer Institute 80: 188–194
46. Dionisi O, Galeotti T, Terranova T, Azzi A 1975 Superoxide radicals and hydrogen peroxide formulation in mitochondria from normal and neoplastic tissues. Biochimica et Biophysica Acta 403: 292–300
47. Barber AA, Wilbur KM 1959 The results of X-irradiation on the antioxidant activity of mammalian tissues. Radiation Research 10: 167–175
48. Gerber M, Richardson S, Salkeld R, Chappuis P 1991 Antioxidants in female breast cancer patients. Cancer Investigations 9(4): 421–428
49. Bartoli GM, Bartoli S, Galeoti T, Bertoli E 1980 Superoxide dismutase content and microsomal lipid composition of tumours with different growth rates. Biochimica et Biophysica Acta 620: 205–211
50. Burns CP, Spector AA 1987 Membrane fatty acid modification in tumour cells: a potential therapeutic adjunct. Lipids 22: 178–184
51. Wood CB, Habib NA, Thompson A, et al 1985 Increase in oleic acid in erythrocytes associated with malignancies. British Medical Journal 291: 163–165.
52. Diplock AT, Balasubramanian K, Manohar M, et al 1988 Purification and chemical characterisation of the inhibitor of lipid peroxidation from intestinal mucosa. Biochimica et Biophysica Acta 962: 42–50
53. Slater TF, Chessman KH, Proudfoot K 1934 Free radicals, lipid peroxidation and cancer. In: Slater TF (ed) Free radicals in molecular biology, aging and disease. Raven Press, New York
54. Eggens I, Backman L, Jakobson A, Valtersson C 1988 The lipid concentration of highly differentiated human hepatomas, with special reference to fatty acids. British Journal of Pathology 69: 671–683
55. Roos DS, Choppin PW 1984 Tumorigenicity of cell lines with altered lipid composition. Proceedings of the National Academy of Sciences, USA 81: 7622–7626
56. Roos DS, Choppin PW 1985 Biochemical studies on cell fusion. I. Lipid composition of fusion resistant cells. Journal of Cell Biology 101: 1578–1590
57. Roos DS, Choppin PW 1985 Biochemical studies on cell fusion. II. Control of cell fusion by lipid alteration. Journal of Cell Biology 101: 1591–1598
58. Dunbar LM, Bailey JM 1975 Enzyme deletions and essential fatty acid metabolism in cultured cells. Journal of Biological Chemistry 250: 1152–1154
59. Bayley JM 1977 Lipid metabolism in cultured cells. In: Snyder F (ed) Lipid metabolism in mammals. Plenum Press, New York, 352–364
60. Chiappe LE, De Tomas ME, Mercuri O 1974 In vitro activity of delta-6 and delta-9-desaturase in hepatomas of different growth rates. Lipids 9: 489–490
61. Howard BV, Howard WJ 1974 Lipid metabolism in cultured cells. Advances in Lipid Research 12: 52–96
62. De Alaniz MJT, Ponz G, Brenner RR 1975 Biosynthesis of desaturated fatty acids in cultured minimal deviation hepatoma 7288c cells. Acta Physiologica et Pharmacologica Latinoamericana 25: 1–11
63. Reitz RC, Thompson HA, Morris HP 1977 Mitochondrial and microsomal phospholipids of Morris hepatoma 7777. Cancer Research 37: 561–567
64. Maeda M, Doi O, Akamatsu Y 1978 Metabolic conversion of polyunsaturated fatty

acids in mammalian cultured cells. Biochimica et Biophysica Acta 530: 153–164

65.   Morton RE, Hartz JW, Reitz RC 1979 The acyl-CoA desaturases of microsomes from rat liver and the Morris 7777 hepatoma. Biochimica et Biophysica Acta 573: 321–331

66.   De Antueno RJ, Niedfield G, De Tomas ME 1988 Microsomal fatty acid desaturation and elongation in a human lung carcinoma grown in nude mice. Biochimica International 16: 413–420

67.   Chapkin RS, Hubbard NE, Buckman DK, Erikson KL 1989 Linoleic acid metabolism in metastatic and nonmetastatic murine mammary tumour cells. Cancer Research 49: 4724–4728

68.   Iturralde M, Gonzalez B, Pineiro A 1990 Linoleate and linolenate desaturation by rat hepatoma cells. Biochimica International 20(1): 37–43

69.   Lynch RD, Locicero J, Schneeberger EE 1986 Metabolism and incorporation into glycerolipids of exogenous 18:3(n–3) and 18:(n–6) by MDCK cells. Lipids 21: 447–453

70.   Bandyopadhyay GK, McKenzie K, Imagawa W, Nandi S 1989 Docosahexaenoic acid is neither synthesized nor retroconverted by the normal and tumour mouse mammary epithelial cells in primary culture. Biochemical and Biophysical Research Communications 158(3): 730–736

71.   Fujiyama-Fujiwara Y, Ohmori C, Igarashi O 1989 Metabolism of gamma-linolenic acid in primary cultures of rat hepatocytes and in Hep G2 cells. Journal of Nutritional Science and Vitaminology 35: 597–611

72.   Nassar BA, Das UN, Huang Y-S, et al 1992 The effect of chemical hepatocarcinogenesis on liver phospholipid composition in rats fed n–6 and n–3 fatty acid-supplemented diets. Chemical Hepatocarcinogenesis 199: 365–368

73.   Schroeder F, Gardiner JM 1984 Membrane lipids and enzymes of cultured high- and low-metastatic B16 melanoma variants. Cancer Research 44: 3262–3269

74.   Calorini L, Fallani A, Tombaccini D, et al 1987 Lipid composition of cultured B16 melanoma cell variants with different lung-colonizing potential. Lipids 22: 651–656

75.   Dahiya R, Yoon W-H, Boyle B, et al 1992 Biochemical, cytogenetic, and morphological characteristics of human primary and metastatic prostate cancer cell lines. Biochemica International 27(4): 567–577

76.   Calderon RO, Grogan WM, Collins JM 1991 Membrane structural dynamics of plasma membranes of living human prostatic carcinoma cells differing in metastatic potential. Experimental Cell Research 196: 192–197

77.   Lanson M, Bougnoux P, Besson P, Lansac J, Hubert B, Covet C, le Floch O 1990 n-6 polyunsaturated fatty acids in human breast cancer carcinoma phosphatidylethanolamine and early relapse. British Journal of Cancer 61: 776–778

78.   Horrobin DF, 1980 The reversibility of cancer: the relevance of cyclic AMP, calcium, essential fatty acids and prostaglandin E_1. Medical Hypotheses 6: 469–486

79.   Dippenaar N, Booyens J, Fabri D, et al 1982 The reversibility of cancer: evidence that malignancy in human hepatoma cells is gamma-linolenic acid deficiency dependent. South African Medical Journal 62: 683–685

80.   Dippenaar N, Booyens J, Fabri D, et al 1982 The reversibility of cancer: evidence that malignancy in melanoma cells is gamma-linolenic acid deficiency dependent. South African Medical Journal 62: 505–509

81.   Booyens J, Dippenaar N, Fabri D 1984 The effect of the prostaglandin precursor gamma-linolenic acid on the rate of proliferation of human osteogenic sarcoma and oesophageal carcinoma cells in culture. South African Medical Journal 65: 240–242

82.   Leary WP, Robinson KM, Booyens J, et al 1982 Some effects of gamma-linolenic acid on cultured human oesophageal carcinoma cells. South African Medical Journal 62: 681–683

83.   Booyens J, Louwrens C, Engelbrecht P 1984 Some effects of the prostaglandin precursor fatty acid, gamma-linolenic acid, and prostaglandin E_1 on the proliferation of human hepatoma cells in culture. South African Medical Journal 60: 144

84.   Girao LA, Cantrill RC, Rock AC, Davidson BC 1987 The influence of C18 fatty acids on the growth of a 3T6 derived cell line. Anticancer Research 7: 133–138

85.   Begin ME, Ells G, Das UN, Horrobin DF 1986 Differential killing of human carcinoma cells supplemented with n-3 and n-6 polyunsaturated fatty acids. Journal of National Cancer Institute 77: 1053–1062

86. Schauenstein E 1967 Autoxidation of polyunsaturated esters in water: chemical structure and biological activity of the products. Journal of Lipid Research 8: 417–428
87. Tolnai S, Morgan JF 1962 Studies on the in vitro antitumor activity of fatty acids v unsaturated acids. Canadian Journal of Biochemical Physiology 40: 869–875
88. Begin ME 1987 Effects of polyunsaturated fatty acids and of their oxidation products on cell survival. Chemistry and Physics of Lipids 45: 269–313
89. Fujiwara F, Todo S, Imashuku S 1984 Antitumor effect of gamma-linolenic acid on cultured human neuroblastoma cells. Prostaglandins Leukotrienes and Medicine 15: 15–34
90. Begin ME, Das UN, Ells G 1986 Cytotoxic effects of essential fatty acids in mixed cultures of normal and malignant human cells. Progress in Lipid Research 25: 573–576
91. Botha JH, Robinson KM, Leary WP 1985 The response of breast carcinoma cell lines to gamma-linolenic acid with special reference to the effects of agents which influence prostaglandin and thromboxane synthesis. Prostaglandins Leukotrienes and Medicine 19: 63–67
92. Booyens J, Engelbrecht P, Le Roux S, et al 1984 Some effects of the essential fatty acids linoleic acid and alpha-linolenic acid and of their metabolites gamma-linolenic acid, arachidonic acid, eicosapentaenoic acid, and docosahexaenoic acid, and of prostaglandins A_1 and E_1 on the proliferation of human osteogenic sarcoma cells in culture. Prostaglandins Leukotrienes and Medicine 15: 15–33
93. Begin ME, Ells G, Das UN 1986 Selected fatty acids as possible intermediates for selective cytotoxic activity of anticancer agents involving oxygen radicals. Anticancer Research 6: 291–296
94. Begin ME, Ells G 1987 Effects of C_{18} fatty acids in breast carcinoma cells in culture. Anticancer Research 7: 215–218
95. Begin ME, Ells G, Horrobin DF 1987 Effects of eicosanoid precursors on TBA reactive material in normal and malignant cells. In: Walden TL, Hughes HN (eds) Prostaglandin and lipid metabolism in radiation injury. Plenum, New York, 345–352
96. Das UN, Begin ME, Ells G, et al 1987 Polyunsaturated fatty acids augment free radical generation in tumor cells in vitro. Biochemical and Biophysical Research Communications 145: 15–24
97. Botha JH, Robinson KM, Ramchurren N, Norman RJ 1989 The role of prostaglandins in the inhibition of cultured carcinoma cell growth produced by gamma-linolenic acid. Prostaglandins Leukotrienes and EFAs 35: 119–123
98. Hayashi Y, Fukushima S, Hirata T, et al 1990 Anticancer activity of free gamma-linolenic acid and the effects of serum albumin an anticancer activity of gamma-linolenic acid in vitro. Journal of Pharmacobio-Dynamics 13: 705–711
99. Mengeaud V, Nano JL, Fournel S, Rampal P 1992 Effects of eicosapentaenoic acid, gamma-linolenic acid and prostaglandin E_1 on three human colon carcinoma cell lines. Prostaglandins Leukotrienes and EFAs 47: 313–319
100. Howie A, Huang Y-S, Horrobin DF 1992 Effects of cholesterol on viability and (n-6) fatty acid metabolism in cultured human monocyte-like cells. Biochemistry and Cell Biology 70: 643–649
101. Ramesh G, Das UN, Koratkar R, et al 1992 Effect of essential fatty acids on tumor cells. Nutrition 8(5): 343–347
102. Sagar PS, Das UN, Koratkar R, Ramesh G, Kumar GS 1992 Cytotoxic action of cis-unsaturated fatty acids on human cervical carcinoma (HeLa) cells: relationship to free radicals and lipid peroxidation and its modulation by calmodulin antagonists. Cancer Letters 63: 189–198
103. Burns CP, Spector AA 1990 Effects of lipids on cancer therapy. Nutrition Review 48: 233–240
104. Burns CP, North JA 1986 Adriamycin transport and sensitivity in fatty acid modified leukemia cells. Biochimica et Biophysica Acta 888: 10–17
105. Burns CP 1988 Membranes and cancer chemotherapy. Cancer Investigations 6: 439–451
106. Chow SC, Sisfontes L, Bjorkhem I, Jondal M 1989 Suppression of growth in a leukemic T cell line by n-3 and n-6 polyunsaturated fatty acid. Lipids 24(8): 700–704
107. Canuto RA, Biocca ME, Muzio G, Dianzani MU 1987 Effect of arachidonic acid on

lipid peroxidation in microsomes of AH-130 hepatoma. Medical Science 15: 1253

108. Takeda S, Horrobin DF, Sim G, Sanford T 1993 GC-MS and UV-spectrophotometric investigation of accelerated lipid peroxidation and cell destruction in cultured human breast cancer cells (ZR-75-1) produced by gamma-linolenic acid and iron. Japanese Journal of Inflammation 13: 27–34

109. Takeda S, Horrobin DF, Manku MS 1992 The effects of gamma-linolenic acid on human breast cancer cell killing, lipid peroxidation and the production of Schiff-reactive materials. Medical Science Research 20: 203–205

110. Takeda S, Horrobin DF, Manku MS, et al 1992 Lipid peroxidation in human breast cancer cells in response to gamma-linolenic acid and iron. Anticancer Research 12: 329–334

111. Takeda S, Sim PG, Horrobin DF, et al 1992 Intracellular free fatty acid release and lipid peroxidation in cultured human breast cancer cells in response to gamma-linolenic acid with iron (GLA + Fe). International Journal of Oncology 1: 759–763

112. Matsuzaki A, Shimura H, Okuda A, et al Mechanism of selective killing by dilinoleoylglycerol of cells transformed by the EIA gene of adenovirus type 12. Cancer Research 49: 5702–5707

113. Anel A, Naval J, Desportes P, et al 1992 Increased cytotoxicity of polyunsaturated fatty acids on human tumoral B and T-cell lines compared with normal lymphocytes. Leukemia 6(7): 680–688

114. Canuto RA, Muzio G, Biocca ME, Dianzani MU 1991 Lipid peroxidation in rat AH-130 hepatoma cells enriched in vitro with arachidonic acid. Cancer Research 51: 4603–4608

115. Peterson DA, Mehta N, Butterfield J, et al 1988 Polyunsaturated fatty acids stimulate superoxide formation in tumor cells: a mechanism for specific cytotoxicity and a model for tumor necrosis factor? Biochemical and Biophysical Research Communications 155(2): 1033–1037.

116. Das UN, Huang Y-S, Begin ME, et al 1987 Uptake and distribution of *cis*-unsaturated fatty acids and their effect on free radical generation. Free Radicals in Biology and Medicine 3: 9–14

117. Takeda S, Sim PG, Horrobin DF, Sanford T, Chisholm K, Simmons V 1993 Mechanism of lipid peroxidation in cancer cells in response to gamma-linolenic acid analyzed by GC-MS (1): conjugated dienes with peroyl (or hydroperoxyl) groups and cell killing effects. Anticancer Research 13: 193–200

118. Sircar A, Cai F, Begin ME, Weber JM 1990 Transformation renders MDR cells more sensitive to polyunsaturated fatty acids. Anticancer Research 10: 1783–1786

119. Begin ME, Sircar S, Weber JM 1994 Differential sensitivity of tumorigenic and genetically related non-tumorigenic cells to cytotoxic polyunsaturated fatty acids. In press

120. Reich R, Royce L, Martin GR 1989 Eicosapentaenoic acid reduces the invasive and metastatic activities of malignant tumor cells. Biochemical and Biophysical Research Communications 160(2): 559–564

121. Spector AA, Burns CP 1987 Biological and therapeutic potential of membrane lipid modification in tumours. Cancer Research 47: 4529–4537

122. Guffy MM, North JA, Burns CP 1984 Effect of cellular fatty acid alteration on adriamycin sensitivity in cultured L1210 murine leukemia cells. Cancer Research 44: 1863–1866

123. Timmer-Bosscha H, Hospers GAP, Meijer C, et al 1989 Influence of docosahexaenoic acid on cisplatin resistance in a human small cell lung carcinoma cell line. Journal of National Cancer Institute 81(14): 1069–1075

124. Zijlstra JG, De Vries EGE, Muskeit FAJ, et al 1987 Influence of docosahexaenoic acid in vitro on intracellular adriamycin concentrations in lymphocytes and human adriamycin-sensitive and resistant small-cell lung cancer cell lines, and on cytotoxicity in the tumor cell lines. International Journal of Cancer 40: 850–856

125. Burns CP, North JA, Petersen ES, Ingraham LM 1988 Subcellular distribution of doxorubicin: comparison of fatty acid-modified and unmodified cells (42760). Proceedings of the Society for Experimental Biology and Medicine 188: 455–460

126. Halmos T, Moroni P, Antonakis K, Uriel J 1992 Fatty acid conjugates of 2′-deoxy-5-fluorouridine as prodrugs for the selective delivery of 5-fluorouracil to tumor cells.

Biochemical Pharmacology 44(1): 149–155

127. Ikushima S, Fujiwara F, Todo S, Imashuku S 1981 Effects of polyunsaturated fatty acids on vincristine-resistance in human neuroblastoma cells. Anticancer Research 11: 1215–1220

128. Sasaki T, Tsukada Y, Deutsch HF, et al 1984 Daunomycin-arachidonic acid complex as a potential new anti-tumor agent. Cancer Chemotherapy and Pharmacology 13: 75–77

129. Chandrabose KA, Cuatrecasas P, Pottathil R, Lang DJ 1981 Interferon-resistant cell line lacks cyclo-oxygenase activity. Science 212: 329–331

130. Pottathil R, Chandrabose KA, Cuatrecasas P, Lang DJ 1980 Establishment of the interferon-mediated antiviral state: role of fatty acid cyclo-oxygenase. Proceedings of the National Academy of Sciences of the USA 77: 5437–5440

131. Hannigan GE, Williams BRG 1991 Signal transduction by interferon-alpha through arachidonic acid metabolism. Science 251: 204–207

132. Furlong ST, Hednis A, Remold HG 1992 Interferon-gamma stimulates lipid metabolism in human monocytes. Cellular Immunology 143: 108–117

133. Farrar WL, Humes JL 1985 The role of arachidonic acid metabolism in the activities of interleukin 1 and 2. Journal of Immunology 135: 1153–1159

134. Santoli D, Phillips PD, Colt TL, Zurier RB 1990 Suppression of interleukin-2-dependent human T cell growth in vitro by prostaglandin E and their precursor fatty acids. Journal of Clinical Investigation 85: 424–432

135. Chang DJ, Ringold GM, Heller RA 1992 Cell killing and induction of manganese superoxide dismutase by tumour necrosis factor is mediated by lipoxygenase metabolites of arachidonic acid. Biochemical and Biophysical Research Communications 188: 538–546

136. Hoeck WG, Ramesha CS, Chang DJ, Fan N, Heller RA, 1993 Cytoplasmic phospholipase A_2 activity and gene expression are stimulated by tumour necrosis factor: doxamethasone blocks the induced synthesis. Procedings of the National Academy of Sciences of the USA 90: 4475–4479

137. Furlong ST, Mednis A, Remold HG 1992 Interferon-gamma stimulates metabolism in human monocytes. Cellular Immunology 143: 108–117

138. Das UN, Ells G, Begin ME, Horrobin DF 1986 Free radicals as possible mediators of the actions of interferon. Journal of Free Radicals in Biology & Medicine 2: 183–188

139. Brekke O-L, Espevik T, Bardal T, Bjerve KS 1992 Effects of n-3 and n-6 fatty acids on tumor necrosis factor cytotoxicity in WEH1 fibrosarcoma cells. Lipids 27(3): 161–168

140. Ladha S, Kingston CA, Bowler K, Manning R 1989 Effect of fatty acid supplementation on the thermal sensitivity of HTC cells in culture. Biochemical Society Transactions 17: 539–541

141. Horrobin DF 1986 The role of essential fatty acids and prostaglandins in breast cancer. In: Reddy BS (ed) Diet, nutrition and cancer: a critical evaluation, Vol 1. CRC Press, Boca Raton, pp 101–124

142. Willett WC, Stampfer MJ, Colditz GA, et al 1987 Dietary fat and the risk of breast cancer. New England Journal of Medicine 316: 22–28

142a. Vatten LJ, Bjerve KS, Anderson A, Jellum E 1993 Polyunsaturated fatty acids in serum phospholipids and risk of breast cancer: a case-controlled study from the Janus serum bank in Norway. European Journal of Cancer 29A: 532–538

142b. Zarides DG, Chevchenko VE, Levtshuk AA, Lifanova YE, Maximovitch DM 1990 Fatty acid composition of erythrocyte membranes and risk of breast cancer. International Journal of Cancer 45: 807–810

142c. Bordoni A, Hrelia S, Biagi PL, Berra B 1992 Different fatty acid profiles in phosphoinositides from human fibroblastic meningiomas with or without chromosome 22 monosomy. International Journal of Cancer 50: 402–404

142d. Chaudry A, McClinton S, Moffatt LEF, Wahle KWJ 1991 Essential fatty distribution in the plasma and tissue phospholipids of patients with benign and malignant prostatic disease. British Journal of Cancer 64: 1157–1160

143. Karmali RA, Donner A, Gobel S, Shimamura T 1980 1. Effect of n-3 and n-6 fatty acids on 7,12-dimethylbenz(a)anthracene-induced mammary tumorigenesis. Anticancer Research 9: 1461–1468

144. Adams LM, Trout JR, Karmali RA 1990 Effect of n-3 fatty acids on spontaneous and experimental metastasis of rat mammary tumour 13763. British Journal of Cancer 61: 290–291

145. Kort WJ, Weijma IM, Bijma AM, et al 1987 Omega-3 fatty acids inhibiting the growth of a transplantable rat mammary adenocarcinoma. Journal of the National Cancer Institute 79(3): 593–599

146. Beck SA, Smith KL, Tisdale MJ 1991 Anticachectic and antitumor effect of eicosapentaenoic acid and its effect on protein turnover. Cancer Research 51: 6089–6093

147. Sakaguchi M, Rowley S, Kane N, et al 1990 Reduced tumour growth of the human colonic cancer cell lines COLO-320 and HT-29 in vivo by dietary n-3 lipids. British Journal of Cancer 62: 742–477

148. De Bravo MG, De Antueno RJ, Toledo J, et al 1991 Effects of eicosapentaenoic and docosahexaenoic acid concentrate on a human lung carcinoma grown in nude mice. Lipids 26(11): 866–870

149. Borgesson CE, Pardini L, Pardini RS, Reitz RC 1989 Effects of dietary fish oil on human mammary carcinoma and on lipid-metabolizing enzymes. Lipids 24(4): 290–295

150. Gonzalez M J, Schemmel R A, Gray J I, et al 1991 Effect of dietary fat on growth of MCF-7 and MDA-MB231 human breast carcinomas in athymic nude mice: relationship between carcinoma growth and lipid peroxidation product levels. Carcinogenesis 12(7): 1231–1235

151. Reissers D, Martin M S, Hammann A, Savadogo A 1991 Effect of fish-containing diet on chemically-induced colon carcinogenesis in rats. Cancer Journal 4(1): 55–57

152. Sobajima T, Tamiya-Koiumi K, Ishihara H, Kojima K 1986 Effects of fatty acid modification of ascites tumor cells on pulmonary metastasis in rat. Japanese Journal of Cancer Research (Gann) 77: 657–663

153. Welsch C 1992 Relationship between dietary fat and experimental mammary tumorigenesis: a review and critique. Cancer Research 52: 2040–2048

154. Ghayur T, Horrobin D F 1981 Effects of essential fatty acids in the form of evening primrose oil on the growth of the rat R3230AC transplantable mammary tumour. IRCS Journal of Medical Science 9: 582

155. Karmali R A, Marsh J, Fuchs C 1985 Effects of dietary enrichment with gamma-linolenic acid upon the growth of the R3230AC mammary adenocarcinoma. Journal of Nutrition Growth and Cancer 2: 41–51

156. Abou El-Ela S H, Prasse K W, Carroll R, Bunce O R 1987 Effects of dietary primrose oil on mammary tumorigenesis induced by 7,12-dimethylbenz(a)anthracene. Lipids 22: 1041–1044

157. Abou El-Ela S H, Prasse K W, Carroll R, et al 1988 Eicosanoid synthesis in 7,12-dimethylbenz(a)anthracene-induced mammary carcinomas in Sprague–Dawley rats fed primrose oil, menhaden oil, or corn oil diet. Lipids 23: 948–954

158. Lee J H, Sugano M 1986 Effects of linoleic and gamma-linolenic acid on 7,12-dimethylbenz(a)anthracene-induced rat mammary tumors. Nutrition Reports International 34: 1041–1049

159. Ramchurren N, Botha J H, Leary W P 1985 An investigation into the effects of gamma-linolenic acid on murine sarcoma M52B. South African Journal Science 81: 331

160. Gardiner N S, Duncan J R 1990 Effect of dietary polyunsaturated fatty acid and d-alpha-tocopherol manipulation on murine melanoma growth. Medical Science Research 18: 923

161. Gardiner N S, Duncan J R 1990 Influence and interactions of polyunsaturated fatty acids and ascorbic acid on murine melanoma growth. Medical Science Research 18: 759

162. Pritchard G A, Jones D L, Mansel R E 1989 Lipids in breast carcinogenesis. British Journal of Surgery 76: 1069–1073

163. Pritchard G A, Mansel R E 1990 The effects of essential fatty acids on the growth of breast cancer and melanoma. In: Horrobin D F (ed) Omega-6 essential fatty acids: pathophysiology and roles in clinical medicine. Alan R Liss, New York, 379–390

164. Nicholson M L, Neoptolemos J P, Clayton H A, et al 1990 Inhibition of experimental

colorectal carcinogenesis by dietary n-6 polyunsaturated fats. Carcinogenesis 11(12): 2191–2197

165. Potworowski E, Bischoff P, Oth D 1992 Prolongation of survival in retrovirally induced T cell lymphoma by dietary omega-6 fatty acid. Nutrition and Cancer 17: 217–221

166. Monis B, Eynard A R 1982 Abnormal cell proliferation and differentiation and urothelial tumorigenesis in essential fatty acid deficient rats. Progress in Lipid Research 20: 691–703

167. Kort W J, Hulsman L O M, Weijma I M, et al 1986 Influence of the linoleic acid content of the diet on tumor growth in transplantable rat tumor models. Annals of Nutrition and Metabolism 30: 120–128

168. Norman A, Bennett L R, Mead L R, Iwamoto K S 1982 Antitumor activity of sodium linolenate. Nutrition and Cancer 11: 107–115

169. McIlmurray M B, Turkie W 1987 Controlled trial of gamma-linolenic acid in Duke's C colorectal cancer. British Medical Journal 294: 1260

170. Van der Merwe C F, Booyens J, Katzeff I E 1987 Oral gamma-linolenic acid in 21 patients with untreatable malignancy. British Journal of Clinical Practice 41: 907–915

2. The effects of eicosapentaenoic acid on tumour growth and cachexia in the MAC16 mouse colon cancer model

M. J. Tisdale

INTRODUCTION

Growth of some tumours is associated with loss of body weight and depletion of adipose tissue and skeletal muscle of the host. This condition, which is referred to as cancer cachexia, depends on the type of the tumour. Thus patients with pancreatic or gastric cancer have the highest frequency of weight loss, whilst patients with breast cancer, acute non-lymphocytic leukaemia and sarcomas have the lowest frequency of weight loss (De Wys 1986). For many tumour types an inverse relationship exists between the degree of weight loss and the median survival time. Even relatively small amounts of weight loss (<5% of body weight) may significantly worsen the prognosis. Although weight loss is observed at an early stage of disease the incidence of weight loss in cancer patients increases with increasing stages of disease (De Wys 1986).

The production of cachexia in cancer patients is obviously complicated by the site of involvement of the tumour, the presence of anorexia and the effect of therapy on food intake. Although anorexia may be present this may not be able to account for the weight loss observed. Thus forced feeding, paired-feeding and caloric restriction experiments in tumour-bearing animals have shown that a decreased food intake alone cannot entirely account for the progressive weight loss (Theologides 1972). In addition clinical studies providing extra calories through total parenteral nutrition (TPN) have failed to prevent the weight loss and in some investigations a decreased survival was observed in the TPN treatment arm (Chlebowski 1985). A number of studies suggest that cancer cachexia is different from simple starvation and that it is due to metabolic abnormalities in addition to the underlying anorexia.

EXPERIMENTAL MODEL

In order to study the complex metabolic situation in cancer cachexia we have utilised a transplantable murine colon adenocarcinoma induced by prolonged administration of 1,2-dimethylhydrazine (Double & Ball 1975). Care must be taken in the selection of appropriate models for the study of cachexia since large tumours may produce effects on the host due to size alone. Thus Morrison et al (1984) showed that an inert artificial tumour depressed host weight gain and skeletal muscle mass up to 30% and food intake up to 20% of that induced by tumours of a comparable size. Cachexia can appear in patients with tumours which are less than 0.01% of the total body weight (Nathanson & Hall 1974) and the total tumour mass in the majority of cancer patients rarely exceeds 0.5 kg.

The MAC16 tumour produces host body weight loss with tumour burdens exceeding 0.3% of the host body weight, and the loss can reach up to 30 to 40% with a tumour burden of only 2.5% (Beck & Tisdale 1987). The reduction in host body weight is directly proportional to the tumour size and is reversible when the tumour is excised (Bibby et al 1987). Weight loss is associated with a depletion of both adipose tissue and skeletal muscle mass without a change in body water content (Table 2.1). Weight loss occurs without a drop in food and water intake (Table 2.1) thus circumventing the complication of anorexia, and providing some indication that the condition may be caused by a circulating catabolic factor produced by the tumour. This material appears to be capable of initiating direct catabolism of adipose tissue and muscle in a manner similar to catabolic hormones (Beck et al. 1990) but appears to be distinct from the cytokines tumour necrosis factor alpha (TNF-α) and interleukin-6 (IL-6) (Mahony et al 1988, Mulligan et al 1992). Although TNF-α is capable of producing weight loss when administered systemically many of the changes appear to differ from those observed in cachectic animals bearing the MAC16 tumour.

Table 2.1   Effect of the MAC16 tumour on food and water intake and body composition of female NMRI mice (mean ± SEM of 9–10 animals per group)

Group	Food intake (Kcal per day)	Water intake (ml per day)	Body water (%)	Body fat (g)	Thigh and gastrocnemius muscle (g)
MAC16 tumour-bearing	8.7 ± 0.7	3.7 ± 0.1	67.6 ± 0.6	0.47 ± 0.10*	0.050 ± 0.005*
Non-tumour-bearing	8.7 ± 0.5	3.8 ± 0.2	69.1 ± 0.8	1.54 ± 0.16	0.065 ± 0.002

*$P<0.01$ from controls using Student's t-test.

Thus in contrast to the absence of anorexia in the MAC16 model the degree of weight loss produced by TNF-α was proportional to a decrease in food and water intake (Mahony et al 1988). While both TNF-α and the MAC16 tumour produced hypoglycaemia and a reduction in the circulatory level of non-esterified fatty acids (NEFA), the effect on the level of plasma triglycerides differed with the MAC16 tumour-induced cachexia causing a decrease and TNF-α producing an increase. No TNF-α was detected in the MAC16 tumour or in the serum of tumour-bearing animals and both tumour and non-tumour-bearing animals responded with a similar elevation of their serum TNF-α levels after endotoxin administration (Mahony et al 1988). In addition monoclonal antibodies specific to TNF-α had no effect on the weight loss in mice bearing the MAC16 tumour (Mulligan et al 1992).

MEDIATORS OF CACHEXIA IN THE MAC16 MODEL

Since loss of adipose tissue occurred early in the process of cachexia induced by the MAC16 tumour and the extent of loss of adipose tissue was proportional to the weight of the tumour, the possibility was considered that the process was initiated by direct catabolism by a tumour factor. To investigate this possibility an in vitro assay was developed employing adipocytes freshly prepared from mouse epididymal adipose tissue and the extent of lipolysis was determined by measuring the release of NEFA or glycerol (Beck & Tisdale 1987). Using such an assay it was found that both extracts of the MAC16 tumour and the serum from weight-losing animals bearing the MAC16 tumour produced an enhanced release of NEFA or glycerol. In contrast the rate of release by two tumours of the MAC series which do not produce cachexia (15A and 13) was less than one-third of that produced by the MAC16 tumour (Beck & Tisdale 1987). In contrast TNF-α had no effect on the mobilization of triglycerides from adipose tissue over a short time period (Mahony et al 1988). The lipid mobilizing activity in the serum of mice bearing the MAC16 tumour varies with weight loss reaching a maximum when the animals had lost 16% of their body weight (Groundwater et al 1990). This suggests that the activity may be required to initiate the cachectic process which is self perpetuating above 16% weight loss. The importance of lipid-mobilizing activity for weight loss is shown in animals bearing the MAC16 tumour, but without weight loss where there is no significant elevation of plasma lipid mobilizing activity above the value found in non-tumour-bearing controls (Groundwater et al 1990).

Further studies have shown that lipid mobilization is induced in animals bearing the MAC16 tumour by a low molecular mass acidic peptide (Beck et al 1990). Material with identical chromatographic and molecular weight characteristics is also present in the serum of patients with cancer cachexia, but is absent from normal serum even under the conditions of starvation. The material is also absent from the serum of patients with Alzheimer's disease and weight loss (Groundwater et al 1990). These results raise the possibility that cachexia in both mice and humans may be initiated by the same material and that this may be tumour specific.

INHIBITION OF THE CACHECTIC PROCESS

If the lipid mobilizing factor is truly responsible for the cachectic state then inhibition of the activity should reverse the cachectic process. Initial studies (Beck & Tisdale 1987) showed that 3-hydroxybutyrate inhibited the enhanced lipid mobilization produced by extracts of the MAC16 tumour in vitro. Ketone bodies have been suggested as directly reducing lipolysis in adipose tissue (Bjorntorp 1966) suggesting that the tumour-produced lipid mobilizing factor was subject to normal metabolic control. In vivo studies showed that when mice bearing the MAC16 tumour were fed a ketogenic diet in which the carbohydrate calories were replaced by fat in the form of medium-chain triglycerides (MCT) host weight loss was prevented with a preservation of both the fat and non-fat carcass mass (Tisdale et al 1987). In addition there was a reduction in the percentage contribution of the tumour to the final body weight. A small patient study showed that a ketogenic diet was also capable of reversing weight loss in cancer patients (Fearon et al 1988). There was, however, no significant alteration in host nitrogen balance or whole body protein synthesis, degradation or turnover rates.

These results, although promising, suggested the need for a more effective inhibitor of the cachectic process. Using the MAC16 model it was observed that diets containing fish oil either with or without MCT significantly reduced host body weight loss, with almost complete protection occurring when the fish oil comprised 50% of the total calories (Tisdale & Dhesi 1990). This effect was observed without an alteration of the total calorie consumption or nitrogen intake. These experiments also showed the fish oil diet to produce a significant reduction in tumour growth rate comparable with that produced by 5-fluorouracil at the maximum tolerated dose. 5-Flurouracil, however, caused almost a doubling of host weight loss while the 50% fish oil diet reversed the weight loss produced by the MAC16 tumour. Since 5-flurouracil is used clinically for the treatment of colonic tumours these results produce some promise for the use of fish oil in the treatment of colonic cancer.

A number of studies have shown n-3 fatty acid diets to be effective inhibitors of the growth of both syngenic and xenografted mammary (Karmali et al 1984), prostatic (Karmali et al 1987) and pancreatic (O'Connor et al 1985) tumours in rodents. In addition a small clinical trial using max EPA capsules as a source of n-3 fatty acids registered a measurable clinical response in two out of 12 heavily pretreated breast cancer patients (Holroyde et al 1988). This study was limited not by toxicity, but by the large number (20) of capsules required to give a sufficient intake of n-3 fatty acids. The dose achievable was 3.6 g eicosapentaenoic acid (EPA) and 2.4 g docosahexaenoic acid (DHA) and the result would warrant further evaluation, using pure fatty acids to enable higher doses to be achieved.

MECHANISM OF ACTION OF LIPID MOBILIZING FACTOR

Lipolysis in adipocytes is thought to be exerted through the intracellular mediator, cyclic AMP, formed in response to activation of adenylate cyclase through binding of the hormone to its receptor (Butcher et al 1968). Studies on the mobilization of triglycerides from epididymal adipocytes in response to the tumour-produced lipid-mobilizing factor showed an elevation of intracellular cyclic AMP (Tisdale & Beck 1991). Moreover, this effect was inhibited by EPA, but not by structurally related fatty acids. This suggests that the active constituent of fish oil is EPA. This was confirmed by in vivo studies in which the administration of pure EPA (95%) to weight-losing mice bearing the MAC16 adenocarcinoma completely reversed and prevented any further decrease in body weight (Fig. 2.1) and inhibited tumour growth (Fig. 2.2). In contrast the other n-

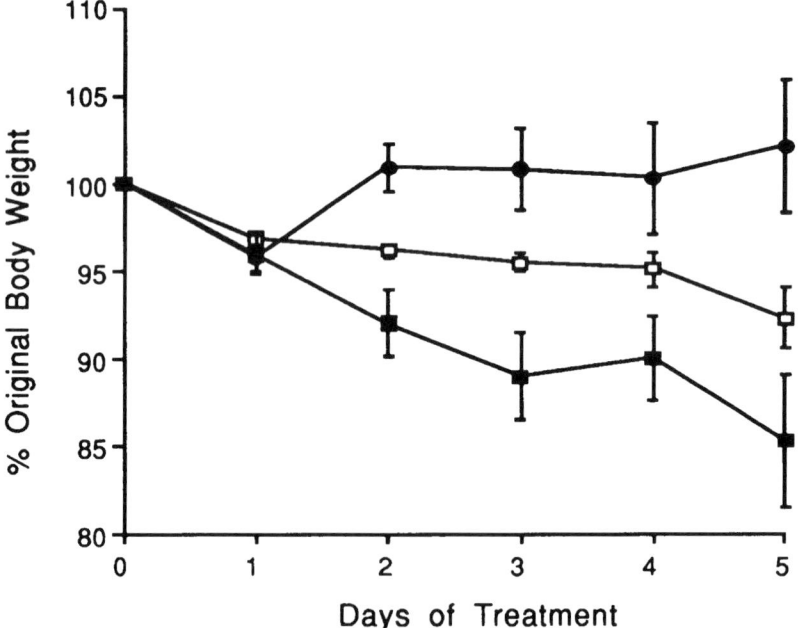

Fig. 2.1   Effect of oral dosing with EPA on the body weight of female mice bearing the MAC16 adenocarcinoma. Mice (20 g) were dosed orally with either 100 μl EPA/d (●), 100 μl linoleic acid/d (■) or 100 μl 0.9% saline/d (□). The experiment was initiated 14 d, after tumour transplantation when weight loss became apparent (average weight loss 5%). Body weights were measured daily and recorded as % maximum body weight attained prior to dosing. Results are expressed as mean ± SEM.

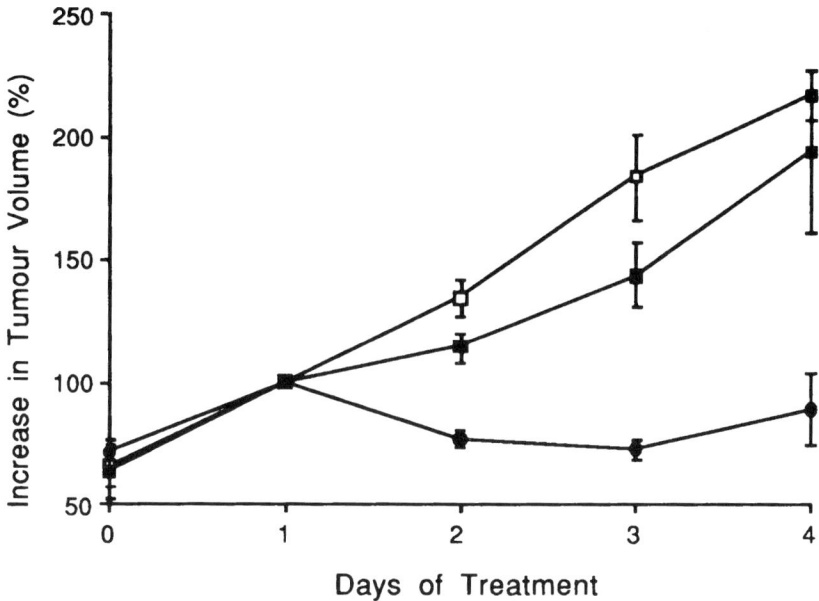

Fig. 2.2 Effect of oral dosing with EPA on the body weight of female mice bearing the MAC16 adenocarcinoma in female NMRI mice. Mice (20 g) were dosed orally with either 100 μl EPA/d (●), 100 μl linoleic acid/d (■) or 100 μl 0.9% saline/d (□). The experiment was initiated 14 d, after tumour transplantation when the tumours became palpable (initial tumour volume = 176 ± 23 mm³). Tumour volumes were measured daily and recorded as % of tumour volume prior to oral dosing. Results are expressed as mean ± SEM.

3 fatty acid present in fish oil, DHA, or the n-6 fatty acid linoleic acid (Figs 2.1 and 2.2) were ineffective in inhibiting weight loss or the growth of the MAC16 tumour.

Preliminary results using plasma membrane fractions of epididymal adipocytes show that lipid-mobilizing factor is capable of direct stimulation of adenylate cyclase and that this effect is inhibited by EPA (Adamson and Tisdale, unpublished results). This suggests that EPA is acting directly at the level of the plasma membrane possibly through the intervention of an inhibitory G-protein (Gi).

In addition to the preservation of adipose tissue, MAC16 tumour-bearing animals treated with EPA also showed retention of skeletal muscle mass. Depletion of skeletal muscle in cachectic mice bearing the MAC16 tumour arises from a small decrease in protein synthesis together with a large increase in protein degradation. Treatment with EPA significantly reduced protein degradation without an effect on protein synthesis (Beck et al 1991). Protein degradation can be achieved in vitro by the addition of serum from weight-losing mice bearing the MAC16 tumour to an isolated gastrocnemius muscle preparation. This suggests the presence of a circulatory factor responsible for degradation of proteins in skeletal muscle, which may be distinct from the lipid-mobilizing factor. Increased protein break-down by the serum factor appears to be associated with an increase in prostaglandin production in gastrocnemius muscle and this effect is inhibited by EPA. The nature of the circulatory factor is unknown but it may be an essential fatty acid such as linoleate or arachidonate which is released from adipose tissue by the tumour lipid-mobilizing factor.

ROLE OF ESSENTIAL FATTY ACIDS (EPA) IN TUMOUR GROWTH

The kinetics of tumour growth inhibition by EPA have been determined using the $[^{125}I]$5-iodo-2′-deoxyuridine method (Gabor et al 1985). This has shown that tumour stasis appears to arise from an increase in the rate of cell loss from 38 to 71% without a significant change in the potential doubling time (Hudson et al 1993). This mechanism of growth inhibition is unusual since most antitumour agents produce tumour growth inhibition by interfering with cell production with consequent effects on the growth of normal tissue compartments with a high turnover rate such as bone marrow, gastrointestinal epithelium, hair follicles and buccal mucosa. This mechanism of growth inhibition may explain the apparent absence of gross toxicity in mice treated with high doses of EPA. The growth of a tumour is a balance between the rate of cell production and the rate of cell loss and for most solid tumours cell production only just exceeds cell loss, so that the doubling time is relatively long (Steel 1977). Thus attempts to increase cell loss may provide a more specific target for therapeutic intervention than interference with cell production.

The antiproliferative, but not the anticachectic, effect of EPA can be reversed by oral administration of pure linoleic acid, which acts to increase tumour growth by reducing the cell loss factor to 45% (Hudson et al 1993). This suggests that EPA may be acting to inhibit tumour growth indirectly by blocking the supply of EFA to the tumour by the inhibition of the tumour-induced lipolysis. There is some data in the literature to suggest that polyunsaturated fatty acids (PUFA), especially of the n-6 series are important determinants in the maintenance of tumour growth. Thus conditions which lead to mobilization of triglycerides from adipose tissue such as an acute fast (Sauer & Dauchy 1987a) and acute streptozotocin-induced diabetes (Sauer & Dauchy 1987b) result in stimulation of tumour growth and the effect appears to be due to uptake of linoleic and arachidonic acids present in hyperlipaemic blood, which appear to be rate limiting for tumour growth in vivo (Sauer & Dauchy 1988).

Linoleic acid has also been shown to stimulate the growth of human breast cancer cell lines in vitro (Rose & Connolly 1989). Cell growth stimulation by linoleic acid appears to be dependent on leukotriene rather than prostaglandin production (Rose & Connolly 1990). The lipoxygenase products may act through cyclic GMP to stimulate cell growth (Buckman et al 1991). Indeed specific arachidonate 5-lipoxygenase inhibitors have been shown to produce potent antiproliferative effects on human leukaemic cell lines in vitro (Tsukada et al 1986) and this may represent an appropriate target for in vivo testing.

In vivo studies using both corn oil and *cis,cis*-linoleic acid showed growth promoting effects against a mouse mammary adenocarcinoma (Hillyard & Abraham 1979). In this case inhibition of prostaglandin synthesis by indomethacin prevented the tumour growth promoting effect. However, care must be taken in the interpretation of the effects of indomethacin, since although at low concentrations it is an inhibitor of prostaglandin synthesis it is also an inhibitor of the lipoxygenase pathway at higher concentrations.

The mechanism for the tumour growth promoting effect of linoleic acid remains unknown. A diverse range of biochemical pathways involved in cellular proliferation entail cleavage of membrane lipids to PUFA which can then act as second messengers (Merrill 1989). In addition adipose tissue has been demonstrated to exhibit angiogenic activity (Silverman et al 1988). Neovascularization is an important determinant for tumour growth in vivo and growth of solid tumours is often limited by an inadequate blood supply. The angiogenic factor has been suggested as 12(R)-hydroxy-eicosatrienoic acid and a metabolite of arachidonic acid via the cytochrome P450-dependent pathway (Masferrer et al 1991).

CONCLUSION

These results suggest that tumour growth is highly dependent on an adequate supply of PUFA and that the process of cachexia, with breakdown of adipose tissue, may be initiated to ensure a continuous supply for tumour growth. EPA is to be considered for clinical investigation and the effective dose based on animal studies has been calculated at between 5 and 10 g per day. This dose is close to the average daily intake (7 g) among Greenland Eskimos and is about twice that previously administered to breast cancer patients as max EPA capsules (Holroyde et al 1988).

ACKNOWLEDGEMENT

This work has been supported by a grant from the Cancer Research Campaign.

REFERENCES

Beck SA, Tisdale MJ 1987 Production of lipolytic and proteolytic factors by a murine tumor producing cachexia in the host. Cancer Research 47: 5919–5923
Beck SA, Mulligan HD, Tisdale MJ 1990 Lipolytic factors associated with murine and human cancer cachexia. Journal of the National Cancer Institute 82: 1922–1926
Beck SA, Smith KL, Tisdale MJ 1991 Anticachectic and antitumour effect of eicosapentaenoic acid and its effect on protein turnover. Cancer Research 51: 6089–6093

Bibby MC, Double JA, Ali SA et al 1987 Characterization of a transplantable adenocarcinoma of the mouse colon producing cachexia in recipient animals. Journal of the National Cancer Institute 78: 539–546

Bjorntorp F 1966 Effect of ketone bodies on lipolysis in adipose tissue *in vitro*. Journal of Lipid Research 7: 621–626

Buckman DK, Hubbard NE, Erickson KL 1991 Eicosanoids and linoleate enhanced growth of mouse mammary tumor cells. Prostaglandins Leukotrienes and Essential Fatty Acids 44: 177–184

Butcher RN, Baird CE, Sutherland EW 1968 Effects of lipolytic and antilipolytic substances on adenosine 3′,5′-monophosphate levels in isolated fat cells. Journal of Biological Chemistry 248: 1705–1710

Chlebowski RT 1985 Critical evaluation of the role of nutritional support with chemotherapy. Cancer 55: 268–272

De Wys WD 1986 Weight loss and nutritional abnormalities in cancer patients: incidence, severity and significance. In: Clinics in oncology. Nutritional support for the cancer patient. 5(2): 251–261

Double JA, Ball CR 1975 Chemotherapy of transplantable adenocarcinoma of the colon in mice. Cancer Chemotherapy Reports 59: 1083–1089

Fearon KCH, Borland W, Preston T et al 1988 Cancer cachexia: influence of systemic ketosis on substrate levels and nitrogen metabolism. American Journal of Clinical Nutrition 47: 42–48

Gabor H, Hillyard LA, Abraham S 1985 Effect of dietary fat on growth kinetics of transplantable mammary adenocarcinoma in BALB/c mice. Journal of the National Cancer Institute 74: 1229–1305

Hillyard LA, Abraham S 1979 Effect of dietary polyunsaturated fatty acids on growth of mammary adenocarcinomas in mice and rats. Cancer Research 39: 4430–4437

Holroyde CP, Skutches CL, Reichard GA 1988 Effect of dietary enrichment with n-3 polyunsaturated fatty acids in metastatic breast cancer. Proceedings of the American Society of Clinical Oncology 7: 42

Hudson EA, Beck SA, Tisdale MJ 1993 Kinetics of the inhibition of tumour growth in mice by eicosapentaenoic acid-reversal by linoleic acid. Biochemical Pharmacology 45: 2189–2194

Karmali RA, Marsh J, Fuchs C 1984 Effect of omega-3 fatty acids on growth of a rat mammary tumor. Journal of the National Cancer Institute 73: 457–461

Karmali RA, Reichel P, Cohen LA et al 1987 The effects of dietary ω-3 fatty acids on the DU-145 transplantable human prostatic tumor. Anticancer Research 7: 1173–1180

Mahony SM, Beck SA, Tisdale MJ 1988 Comparison of weight loss induced by recombinant tumour necrosis factor with that produced by a cachexia-inducing tumour. British Journal of Cancer 57: 385–389

Masferrer JL, Rimarachin JA, Gerritsen ME et al 1991 12(R)-Hydroxyeicosatrienoic acid, a potent chemotactic and angiogenic factor produced by the cornea. Experimental Eye Research 52: 417–424

Merrill AH 1989 Lipid modulators of cell function. Nutrition Reviews 47: 161–169

Morrison SD, Moley JF, Norton JA 1984 Contribution of inert mass to experimental cancer cachexia in rats. Journal of the National Cancer Institute 73: 991–998

Mulligan HD, Mahony SM, Ross JA, Tisdale MJ 1992 Weight loss in a murine cachexia model is not associated with the cytokines tumour necrosis factor-α or interleukin-6. Cancer Letters 65: 239–243

Nathanson L, Hall TC 1974 Lung tumors. How they produce their syndromes. Annals of the New York Academy of Sciences 230: 367–377

O'Connor TP, Roebuck BD, Peterson F, Campbell TC 1985 Effect of dietary intake of fish oil and fish protein on the development of L-azaserine-induced preneoplastic lesions in rat pancreas. Journal of the National Cancer Institute 75: 959–962

Rose DP, Connolly JM 1989 Stimulation of human breast cancer cell lines in culture by linoleic acid. Biochemical and Biophysical Research Communications 164: 277–283

Rose DP, Connolly JM 1990 Effects of fatty acids and inhibitors of eicosanoid synthesis on the growth of a human breast cancer cell line in culture. Cancer Research 50: 7139–7144

Sauer LA, Dauchy RT 1987a Blood nutrient concentrations and tumor growth *in vivo* in rats: relationships during the onset of an acute fast. Cancer Research 47: 1065–1071

Sauer LA, Dauchy RT 1987b Stimulation of tumour growth in adult rats *in vivo* during acute streptozotocin-induced diabetes. Cancer Research 47: 1756–1761

Sauer LA, Dauchy RT 1988 Identification of linoleic and arachidonic acids as the factors in hyperlipemic blood that increase [^{3}H]thymidine incorporation in hepatoma 7288CTC perfused *in situ*. Cancer Research 48: 3106–3111

Steel GG 1977 Growth kinetics of tumours. Cell population kinetics in relation to the growth and treatment of cancer. Clarendon Press, Oxford

Theologides A 1972 Pathogenesis of cachexia in cancer. A review and a hypothesis. Cancer 29: 484–488

Tisdale MJ, Brennan RA, Fearon KC 1987 Reduction of weight loss and tumour size in a cachexia model by a high fat diet. British Journal of Cancer 56: 39–43

Tisdale MJ, Beck SA 1991 Inhibition of tumour-induced lipolysis *in vitro* and cachexia and tumour growth *in vivo* by eicosapentaenoic acid. Biochemical Pharmacology 41: 103–107

Tsukada T, Nakashima K, Shirakawa S 1986 Arachidonate 5-lipoxygenase inhibitors show potent antiproliferative effects on human leukaemia cell lines. Biochemical and Biophysical Research Communications 140: 832–836

3. Effects of gamma-linolenic acid and lithium gamma-linolenate on human hepatoma cells and monocytes

M. C. A. Puntis W. G. Jiang

INTRODUCTION

The ability of a tumour to grow is the net result of a complex interaction of many factors. Metabolic substrates of the right type and in appropriate proportions, which might be different from the requirements of normal cells, must be available for mitosis and growth of the cancer. The tumour must induce the formation of its own neovasculature to maintain a supply of nutrients once it has grown beyond microscopic proportions. A malignant growth, by its very nature, is not subject to the usual cellular growth constraints and grows out of control into and beyond the parent tissue from which it arose. Host defence mechanisms whose normal function is to destroy non-self tissue fail or are fooled into inactivity and allow the malignant cells to grow and invade.

These properties that have evolved in malignant cells to enable the tumour's survival provide us with a few portals through which we might be able to manipulate the tumour cells or introduce agents that will sabotage the otherwise unchecked progress of the cancer. The interaction of monocytes and macrophages with tumour cells may provide a means of control but it is far from completely understood at present. The macrophage holds a central role in the initiation and coordination of the immune system because of its responsibility for antigen presentation (Rosenthal & Shevach 1973, Shevach & Rosenthal 1973) and its ability to modulate so many other processes by the release of a wide range of cytokines and intra-cellular messengers. A current list of the cytokines and growth factors produced by monocyte/macrophage cells is shown in Table 3.1.

Table 3.1.   Cytokines produced by monocyte/macrophage cells

Cytokine	MW kDA	Stimuli	Other sources	Properties
IL-1α & IL-1β*	17	LPS, mit & cytok	Various cells	Immune regulation
IL-3	14–30	WEHI-3 cell	T cells	Haematopoietic
IL-6*	26	LPS, cytok, mito	T, B KT, ET & tumour cells	Haematopoietic, inflamm
IL-8* family	8.5	LPS	ET & tumour cells	Immune regulation, cell growth
IL-10*	18.7	LPS	T cells	Cytokine production
IL-11	20	?	BM & stroma cell	Stimulates haematopoiesis
IL-12*	70	SAC & PMA	B & T cells	NK and T cell stimulation
TGF-β	2×12.5	LPS	Various cells	Cell growth, immune regulation etc
TNFα	3×17.5	LPS, PMA & others	T, PMN, NK & Tumour cells	Cell growth, immune regulation
G-CSF	18–22	LPS, IL-1 & TNF	ET, FB & T cells	Immune regulation, haematopoietic
M-CSF/CSF-1	45–70	PMA & adherence	ET & various cells	Haematopoietic, immune regulation
GM-CSF	22	LPS, PMA & ILs	ET & T cell	Haematopoietic, immune regulation
IGF-I	6	Various	Various cells	Cell growth & motility
PDGF	30–32	LPS & PMA	Various cells	Cell growth & other functions
HGF/SF	69+34	?	FB & fat cells,	Cell growth & motility
IFNα & IFNβ	16–27	LPS & pathogen	B cells	Cell growth and immune regulation
EGF/TGFα	5–20	Various	Various cells,	Cell growth and immune regulation
bFGF	15.6–17.8	?	Various cells	Angiogenesis, cell growth
Activin-A/ Inhibin-βAβA	28	?	Gonadal cells	Hormone release, haemotopoietic
Oncostadin M	28	PMA	T cells	Malignant cell growth inhibition
MIP1α/1β/ RANTES/JE/ LD78/MCP-1*	8	LPS & GM-CSF	T cells	Immune regulation
MIP-2/ platelet factor 4 family*	6	LPS	Platelets	Haematopoietic, immune regulation
HILDA/LIF	38	PMA & VD3	T & tumour cells	Immune responses

* monocyte/macrophage as major contributor in vivo. HILDA: human interleukin for DA cells. LIF: leukemia inhibitory factor

Fatty acids

The fatty acids that we ingest as part of our normal diet are absorbed from the gut and taken up into the tissues, particularly the phospholipids and therefore the composition of the dietary intake of fatty acids affects the proportions of the fatty acids and their metabolites in the tissues (Yang-Yi Fan & Chapkin 1992). Most polyunsaturated fatty acids (PUFA) are esterified to the sn-2 position of phospholipids, from here they can be released by phospholipases and then as free fatty acids form a starting point for a complex biochemical system whereby the fatty acid chain may be de-saturated and elongated to form a family of extremely important and biologically active molecules: the eicosanoids, comprising the leukotrienes, prostaglandins and the thromboxanes.

The three principal groups of fatty acids in mammalian metabolism are defined by the position of the last double bond from the methyl end of the fatty acid chain. Oleic acid (18:1n-9) is the parent substance for the n-9 group, linoleic acid (18:2n-6) for the n-6 family and linolenic (18:3n-3) for the n-3 fatty acid family. The conversion of linoleic to gamma-linolenic acid (18:3n-6) (GLA) and the conversion of linolenic to sterari-donic acid (18:4n-3) share the same rate limiting enzyme, delta-6-desaturase (Δ6d). GLA is the first substance formed beyond this enzyme in the n-6 series. It is of particular relevance to the present sphere of study because malignant cells have been shown to have decreased Δ6d activity (Dunbar & Bailey 1975), the addition of exogenous GLA to tumour cells may overcome this deficiency and enable metabolic pathways that are suppressed in malignant cells to function (Reid et al 1991). These pathways may be to the detriment of the cell. This is therefore important and warrants further study.

GLA is de-saturated further and elongated to arachidonic acid (20:4n-6) which is then converted via the lipoxygenase pathway to the leucotrienes or via the cyclooxygenase pathway to the prostaglandins. The n-3 fatty acids are similarly de-saturated and elongated to eicosapentanoic acid (20:5n-3) which again can enter the lipoxygenase or cyclooxygenase path. Different members of the leukotriene and prostaglandin family are derived from n-3 and n-6 PUFAs. It is by means of these potent and often immune-reactive derivatives that PUFAs exert many of their effects on cells and organ systems and due to the competition for the shared enzyme systems early in the metabolic pathway dietary modification can alter the relative proportions of the pre-cursors and hence of the end products (Yang-Yi Fan & Chapkin 1992).

Role of fatty acids as potential anti-cancer drugs

There is accumulating evidence that fatty acids and especially GLA may have an anti-tumour effect (Das 1990), as it circumvents the Δ6d deficiency of certain tumour cells and allows prostaglandins to form, many of which have anti-tumour properties (Sakai et al 1984)

The content of PUFAs in tumour cells is deficient (Bartoli et al 1980) and the addition of exogenous GLA may help to overcome this. There is also a reduced capacity for free radical generation in tumour cells (Cheeseman et al 1986); this is often triggered by PUFAs (Das et al 1987) as they undergo peroxidation. GLA might restore this mechanism to normal.

There is evidence that the ability of tumour necrosis factor (TNF) and interferon-gamma (IFNγ) to kill cells is PUFA dependent. TNF and IFN may well exert their effect by the activation of phospholipase A2 (PLA2) which will release PUFAs from phospholipids. The fatty acids can trigger oxidative metabolism and hence the release of free radicals in neutrophils and tumour cells. This mechanism might be diminished in tumour cells because of the reduced PUFA content.

The activity of cytotoxic drugs, for example doxorubicin and mitomycin C, involves the release of oxidative radicals. It might well be that the mechanism is via PLA2 releasing PUFAs that subsequently undergo peroxidation to release free radicals. Decreased PLA2 and PUFAs in tumour cells may contribute to cytotoxic drug resistance and this might be reversible by the addition of GLA.

EXPERIMENTAL WORK

We have endeavoured, in a series of in vitro experiments, to discover some of the basic mechanisms which underpin the use of EFAs in the treatment of cancer. The techniques which we have developed and describe here will, we hope, also be of use in monitoring the course of patients in forthcoming clinical trials of GLA in malignant disease.

Our work is in two sections. The first deals with the effect of GLA and its lithium salt (LiGLA) on monocytes. These have be drawn from a population of normal controls and a group of patients with obstructive jaundice, often due to malignant disease. The second section is concerned with the way in which fatty acids can modify the effect of cytokines on the growth of a human hepatoma cell line.

REGULATION OF MONOCYTE FUNCTION BY ESSENTIAL FATTY ACIDS

Patients with obstructive jaundice are known to have disturbed immune function (Holman et al. 1979, Pain 1987, Puntis and Jiang 1992a), which may influence their host response to the tumour that may be the cause of the jaundice and also will contribute to their increased risk of septic complications (Holman et al 1979, Blamey et al 1983, Pain et al 1985, Wait & Kahng 1989). These patients have increased monocyte TNFα and IL-6 production, lysosomal enzyme secretion (Jiang et al 1991, Puntis & Jiang

1992a) and neutrophil oxidative response (Puntis and Jiang 1991). The function of both monocytes and neutrophils has also been shown to have a bearing on patients' immediate clinical outcome (Jiang et al 1992, Puntis & Jiang 1992a,b). Monocyte and neutrophil function in jaundiced patients is similar to that observed in patients with sepsis, adult respiratory distress syndrome (ARDS) and trauma, where monocytes and neutrophils are both activated and may cause damages to the host (Mozes et al 1991, Tanaka et al 1991, Trautinger et al 1991). The occurrence of endotox-aemia in these patients may in part contribute to the activation of the monocyte/macrophage population (Wardle & Wright 1970, Hunt et al 1982). In view of the effects of monocyte activation on the host, clinical intervention to modify the imbalance of immune cell function may be helpful. Anti-endotoxin antibodies (Opal et al 1991, Ziegler et al 1991, Eskandari et al 1992), anti-cytokine antibodies (Fong et al 1989, Starnes et al 1990, Opal et al 1991), cytokine receptor antagonist (Fischer et al 1992), or primer antibodies (Redmond et al 1991, O'Riodain et al 1992) have all been explored in recent years and some of them have been shown to be of limited benefit to some patients, but these agents are expensive, and have side effects which detract from their benefits. There is a need, therefore, to find more economic, safe and physiological means to control the activity of the monocyte/macrophage population in an attempt to try to improve these patients.

The essential fatty acids (EFA) and particularly their metabolites, such as leukotriene B4 are involved in immune regulation (Hwang 1989). There are a few essential fatty acids known to possess immuno-inhibitory effects and these have been used in rheumatoid arthritis (Belch et al 1988), chronic inflammatory diseases (Kunkel et al 1981), and primary cirrhosis (Trigger 1990), in which patients have an immune dysfunction similar to that reported in jaundiced patients (Jiang et al 1991, Puntis and Jiang 1991, Bemelmans 1992, Jiang et al 1992, Puntis & Jiang 1992a, b).

As EFAs have an effect on immune function and there is an EFA deficiency in jaundiced patients (Scriven et al 1992), we hypothesize that the immune function of monocytes from jaundiced patients could be modified and tested by supplementation in vitro with EFAs. In this study we examined the effects of the n-6 fatty acid, GLA and LiGLA on monocyte secretory functions and report here that cells from control and jaundiced patients have different responses to the fatty acids. There is a stimulatory effect on TNFα production in control monocytes and an inhibitory effect on both TNFα and lysosomal enzyme production in monocytes from jaundiced patients.

Experimental methods

Preparation of monocytes

Monocytes from peripheral blood drawn from an antecubital vein were separated by Ficoll–Hypaque centrifugation, and purified by an adherence technique. The monocytes thus obtained were 96% pure as determined by non-specific esterase and endogenous peroxidase staining. All the procedures prior to cell culture were carried out at 4°C to avoid cell activation.

Cell culture conditions

Monocytes were suspended in RPMI 1640 with 5% fetal calf serum (FCS), penicillin and streptomycin. Experiments were conducted in 96-well microtitre plates and included control cells treated with culture medium alone and treatment cells treated with fatty acids at concentrations between 1 and 100 μM. Lithium carbonate was added to some wells as a control for the lithium in LiGLA. Ethanol was used as a solvent for the fatty acids and was present in all cultures.

In order to determine whether the effects of fatty acids on monocytes were due to their metabolites, cells in selected cultures were also treated with nordihydroguaiaretic acid (NDGA) (a lipooxygenase inhibitor), indomethacin (a cyclooxygenase inhibitor) or tocopherol (an antioxidant). The trypan blue exclusion test was used after the culture period to test the viability of the monocytes.

TNF assay

For TNF studies, cells in either control or fatty-acid-containing medium were stimulated with lipopolysaccharide (LPS) at 10 μg/ml for 24 h and the cell free supernatants were then stored at –80°C before being assayed. Tumour necrosis factor alpha (TNFα) was measured by using a standard L929 bioassay (Neale et al 1989). Briefly, L929 cells are seeded onto 96-well plates and left overnight to reach confluence. Monocyte supernatant or recombinant human TNFα (rhTNFα), serially diluted in actinomycin-D medium (final concentration 1.0 μg/ml), is added to the cells. After 23 h culture, cells are fixed and stained with crystal violet. The TNFα activity was quantified against rhTNFα and calculated as U/ml: 1 unit (U) is the concentration of TNFα producing half maximal killing of target cells.

Lysosomal enzyme assay

For lysosomal enzyme studies, cells were cultured for 4 h with or without fatty acids and supernatants were again stored at –80°C.

The secretion of the lysosomal enzyme, β-hexosaminidase, was measured spectrophotometrically by using the specific substrate, nitrophenol-β-D-glu-cosaminide, which is split by the enzyme to produce the coloured product, nitrophenol (Tsao et al 1979, Chatterjee et al 1982) (measured with a Titertek Multiscan). The results are calculated as U/ml: 1 U is the concentration of the enzyme needed to produce 1 μM/min nitrophenol (commercial nitrophenol was used in the experiments as an internal standard).

Results

TNFα and hexosaminidase production by monocytes from normal and jaundiced patients

Cells from jaundiced patients compared with the non-jaundiced controls showed greatly increased TNFα production when stimulated with LPS. The hexosaminidase levels are also raised compared with controls (Fig. 3.1). This suggests that monocytes from jaundiced patients are activated in vivo prior to testing.

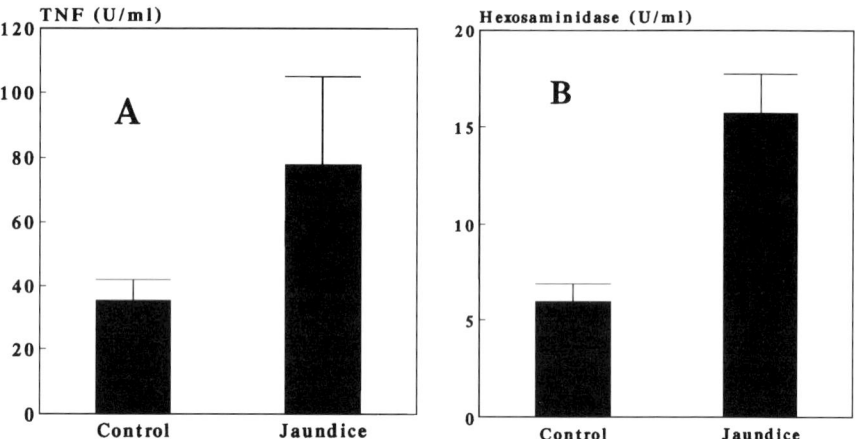

Fig. 3.1.   Monocyte TNF and hexosaminidase production. Cells from jaundiced patients compared with normal controls show (A) significantly increased TNF (LPS stimulated) release and also (B) significantly increased hexosaminidase release. The columns represent means with SEM. Student's t-test, $P<0.01$ taken as significant.

The effects of fatty acid on monocyte TNFα production

When cultured with GLA or LiGLA, monocytes from normal volunteers increased their TNFα production. Lithium carbonate has a small but nevertheless significant effect (Fig. 3.2), and LiGLA has a more profound effect than GLA at concentrations as low as 0.1 μM. The effect of the lithium ions alone is not enough to account for this; the lithium carbonate has an effect which is only seen at its lower concentrations.

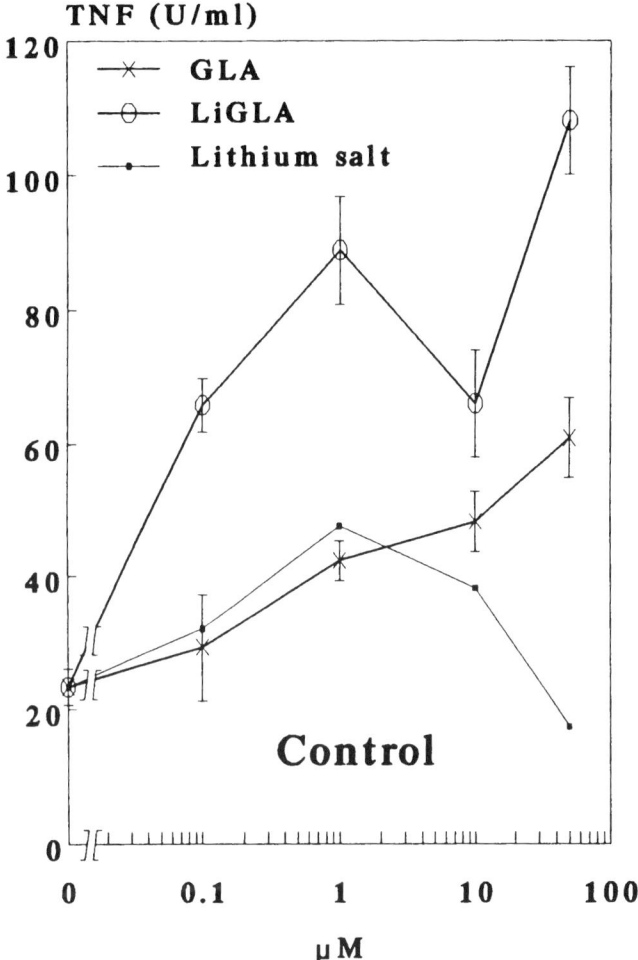

Fig 3.2. Effects of GLAs on TNF production from control monocytes. In control monocytes, lithium salt, GLA, and lithium GLA all increase TNFα production; a much more powerful effect is seen with lithium GLA (LiGLA) than with GLA.

Other fatty acids tests, hexanoic acid, linoleic acid, and arachidonic acid, have no significant effects (data not shown).

Patients with obstructive jaundice have increased levels of TNF production compared with controls and the effect of GLA and LiGLA on monocytes from these patients is strikingly different. TNF production by jaundiced patients' monocytes shows a negative response to treatment with GLA. The fatty acid causes a dose-dependent reduction in TNF production (Fig. 3.3). LiGLA shows a similar degree of inhibition.

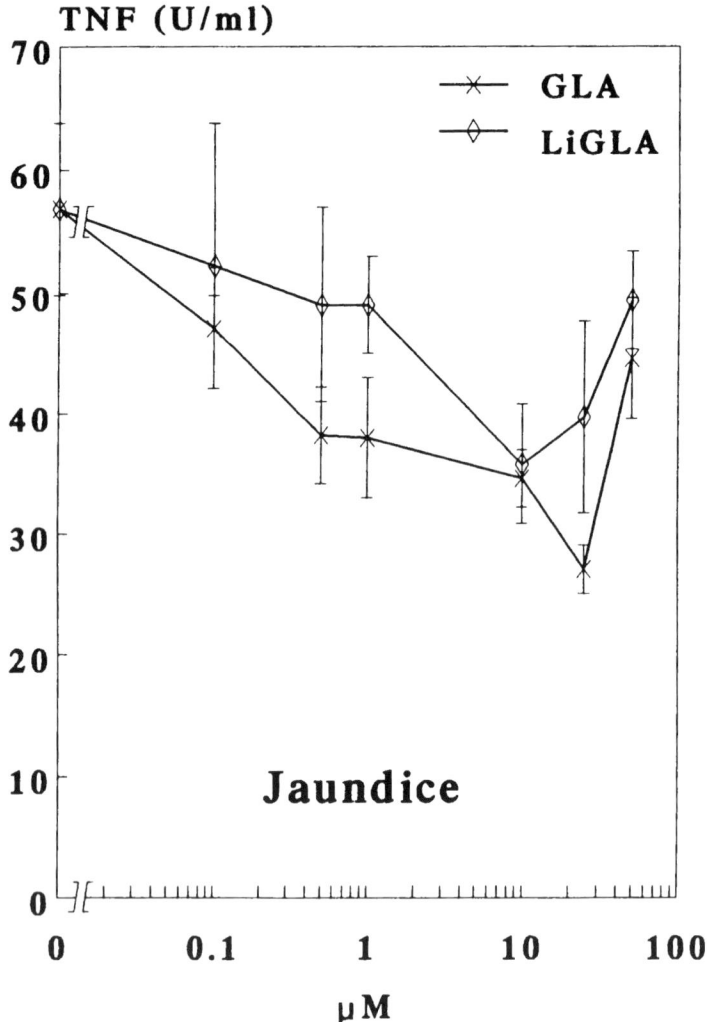

Fig. 3.3. Effects of GLAs on TNF production from jaundiced monocytes. Jaundiced monocytes, which have an increased TNF production, reduce their TNF production in the presence of both forms of GLA.

GLA and LiGLA have similar stimulatory effects on monocytes from both benign and malignant controls (Table 3.2). Inhibitory effects are seen in patients with either benign or malignant jaundice (Table 3.2).

The effects of fatty acids on monocyte β-hexosaminidase secretion

Culture of cells from normal volunteers with GLA produces no significant change; jaundiced cells, however, which usually produce abnormally high levels of β-hexosaminidase are down-regulated by GLA and LiGLA. The secretion levels return toward those seen in controls (Fig. 3.4). This inhibitory effect was seen in patients with both benign and malignant jaundice (data not shown). Lithium carbonate has no significant effects on monocyte β-hexosaminidase secretion from either control or jaundiced patients.

Table 3.2. Monocyte TNFα production in both control and jaundiced patients

	Control		Jaundiced	
	Benign ($n=7$)	Malig ($n=5$)	Benign ($n=6$)	Malig ($n=9$)
Medium	30.0±3.4	20.4±4.0	49.8±2.9	78.2±4.7
GLA(1 μM)	42.3±8.0	42.4±5.3	34.3±5.9	39.5±6.0
GLA (10 μM)	59.5±9.0	62.8±6.4	16.2±4.8	39.6±5.8
LiGLA (1 μM)	65.8±7.2	98.8±8.0	29.9±6.8	40.1±6.3
LiGLA (10 μM)	82.8±5.4	86.0±8.0	39.4±8.2	48.3±4.2

TNF shown as U/ml as assayed by L929 cell bioassay. Both GLA and LiGLA increased the production of TNF from both benign and malignant control, whereas the increased TNF productions from all jaundiced groups are inhibited by GLA and LiGLA.

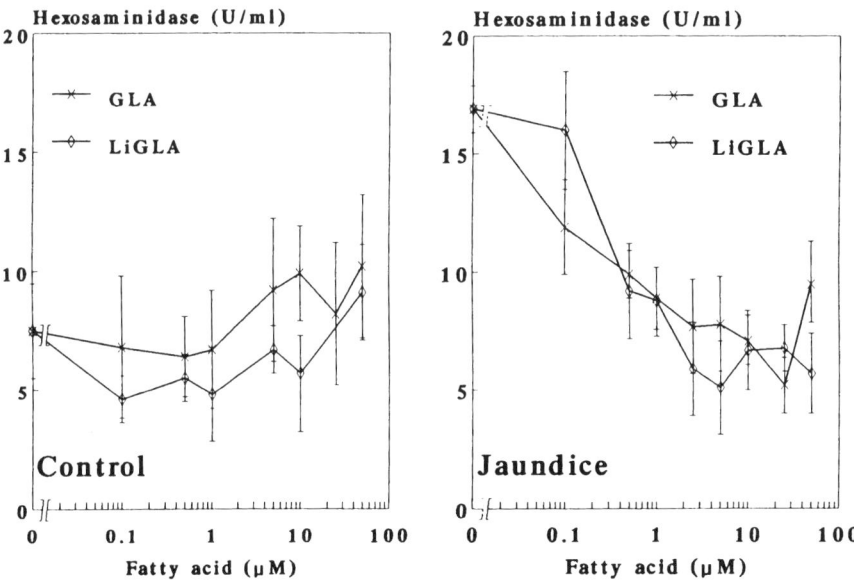

Fig. 3.4. The effects of GLAs on monocyte hexosaminidase production. Neither GLA nor LiGLA has significant effects on the enzyme secretion from control monocytes (left). In contrast, both GLAs have significant inhibitory effects on the hexosaminidase secretion from jaundiced monocytes, which have a significantly higher base level than control monocytes.

The possible involvement of fatty acid metabolites

All experiments included cultures containing inhibitors for lipid metabolism. When monocytes were cultured with GLA in the presence of inhibitors, NDGA (which inhibits lipooxygenase), indomethacin (which inhibits cyclooxygenase), or the antioxidant tocopherol, the response to GLA was found not to be affected in spite of using a wide range of inhibitor concentrations, 1–50 μM (Fig. 3.5). This suggests that the metabolic products of GLA do not play a significant role in GLA-mediated effects on monocytes.

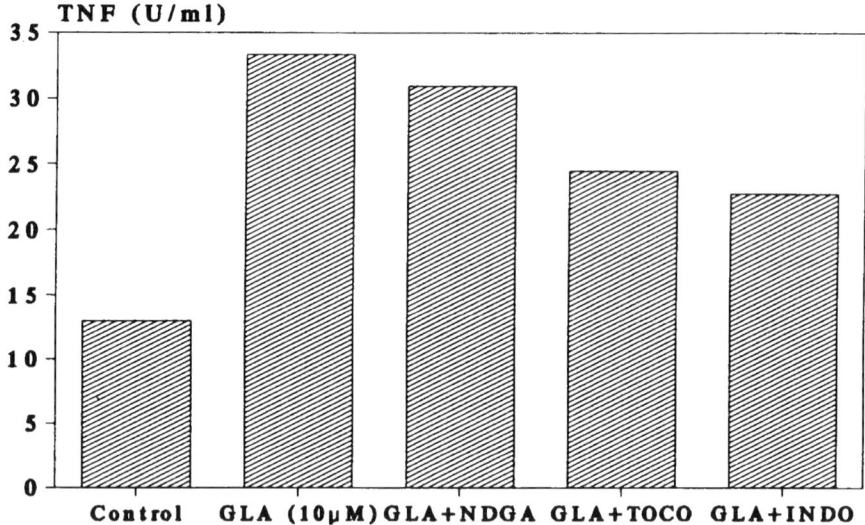

Fig 3.5.   The possible contribution of enzyme inhibitors in GLA induced TNF production. Cells were cultured with GLA (10 μM) with or without NDGA, indomethacin, or tocopherol at 10 μM. There is no significant blocking with the inhibitors. Control cultures are significantly lower than GLA cultures. Student's *t*-test, *P*<0.01 taken as significant.

Monocyte viability

Viability was checked by trypan blue exclusion; there was no difference between control cells and cells cultured with gamma linolenic acid up to 100 μM (Fig. 3.6). This indicates that the inhibitory effects of fatty acids on monocyte functions are not due to cytoxicity.

OVERVIEW

The data outlined above support the contention that the n-6 fatty acid, GLA, may be an important means of modifying immune functions.

Different functional states of the monocytes may account for the various cellular responses seen in the different groups investigated. GLA and

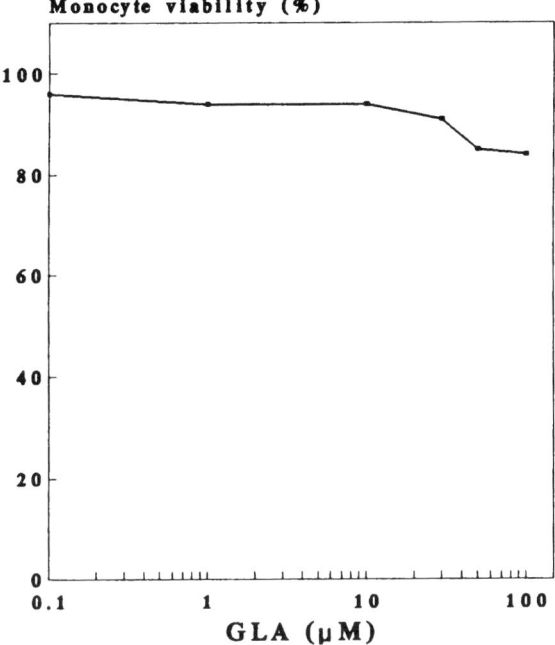

Fig. 3.6. Viability of monocytes cultured with GLA. Viability of monocytes cultured with GLA as measured by trypan blue exclusion. No significant loss of viability is seen with GLA concentrations up to 100 μM.

its lithium salt has up-regulatory effects on TNF production and no effects on hexosaminidase secretion of normal monocytes. However both TNF and hexosaminidase production, which are increased in jaundice, are down-regulated by GLA and LiGLA.

The precise mechanisms of GLA regulation of different monocyte functions are not clear. Although it is suggested that the effects of essential fatty acids on immune cells may be via their metabolites (Hwang, 1989), our data shows that this is probably not so. Inhibiting the enzymes involved in GLA metabolism with NDGA or indomethacin does not influence the effect. The antioxidant tocopherol also has no effect. The inhibitory effect of GLA on monocyte lysosomal enzyme appears only after 4 h culture, implying that some preliminary metabolic activity must first occur. One of GLA's metabolites and the immediate precursor of the eicosanoids, arachidonic acid (AA), has no significant effect on TNF production (data not shown). The viability data (Fig. 3.6) also exclude the possibility of cytoxicity of GLA on monocytes. It is reported that polyunsaturated fatty acids when cultured with cells may quickly be incorporated into cell membranes and thereby modify cell functions (Schroit & Gallily 1979, Mohoney et al. 1980, Lokesh & Wrann 1984, Hagve 1988); a change in GLA levels in monocyte cell membranes could easily modify cell function because of the change in membrane fluidity.

It is reported that lithium salts can potentiate TNF production from monocyte/macrophage cells (Kleinerman et al 1989). We have confirmed that lithium carbonate can increase TNF production, but we have also shown that LiGLA, a water-soluble lithium salt of GLA, has an even greater effect than GLA on the cell, possibly because of the additional effect of increased availability of the fatty acid to the cell.

The responses to fatty acids of cells from normal and jaundiced monocytes are strikingly diffferent. The reasons for this are not yet fully elucidated. The data shown in Fig. 3.1 clearly show that monocytes from jaundiced donors are in an activated state as indicated by increased lysosomal enzyme and TNF release. Renz et al (1988) have reported that macrophages in different functional states may respond differently to PGE_2: resting cells increase their cGMP and TNFα production is up-regulated, activated cells, however, increase their cAMP and TNFα production is down-regulated. Whether this phenomenon is involved in GLA-mediated TNF production remains to be seen. Jaundiced patients have an EFA deficiency (Scriven et al 1992). It is also known that there is a relationship between the saturation of cell membranes and cell function (Hagve 1988); this suggests that monocytes from a jaundiced host may have a different fatty acid pattern, accounting, in part, for the different responses to stimulation seen in these cells (Schroit & Gallity 1979, Mohoney et al 1980).

The potential clinical importance of the effect of GLA on monocytes is obvious. Firstly, there may be a role in the treatment of cancer. It has been reported that patients who bear solid tumours (but are not jaundiced) may have reduced monocyte TNF production and low blood TNF levels (Socher et al 1988, Zielinski et al 1990). Our data clearly shows that in control monocytes, the production of TNF is increased by supplementation with GLA, lithium, or Li GLA. It is also reported that GLA itself is cytotoxic to malignant cells (Horrobin 1990) and that lithium may increase TNF-mediated cytoxicity to cancer cells (Beyaert & Fiers 1992). The use of GLA and its lithium salt may therefore be beneficial, by these multiple mechanisms, in the management of malignant tumours. Patients who have obstructive jaundice, in common with those who have sepsis, trauma, ARDS etc., also have activated monocytes and neutrophils (Jiang et al 1991, Mozes et al 1991, Puntis & Jiang 1991b, Tanaka et al 1991, Trautinger et al 1991, Bemelmans 1992, Jiang et al 1992, Puntis & Jiang 1992a). Hitherto attempts to modify the over-activation of monocytes and other immune cells have concentrated on using various antibodies or stimuli antagonists (Fong et al 1989, Starnes et al 1990, Opal et al 1991, Ziegler et al 1991, Eskandari et al 1992, Fisher et al 1992), and have not been totally satisfactory. Most of these are recombinant or synthetic proteins that are expensive, and often poorly tolerated by patients. The immune cells are activated by a variety of agents in vivo, including endotoxin and cytokines. Blocking a single stimulus or primer will therefore not be enough to prevent the activation or to deactivate the monocyte/macrophage population. Using a fatty acid, however, may overcome some of the disadvantages. It is available in a pharmaceutically approved form and is relatively cheap and safe, although lithium can easily reach toxic levels.

In conclusion, we report here that n-6 fatty acid is a monocyte function regulator. Cells from normal and jaundiced patients have different responses to the fatty acids. This may provide some immunological background for the clinical use of EFAs.

THE REGULATION OF CYTOKINE-INDUCED HEPATOMA CELL GROWTH BY n-6 FATTY ACIDS

Hepatocellular cancer kills between 250 000 and 1 250 000 people each year worldwide. In Nigeria the incidence is 16.4 per 100 000 compared with 2–3 per 100 000 in the west. The hepatitis B virus is a major aetiological factor, many cases being associated with the presence of the hepatitis B surface antigen (HBsAg) in the serum.

In the last few years some cytokines have been shown to be able to control cancer cell growth. A few cytokines have an effect on hepatoma cells, IFNγ, TNFα and most recently HGF, are reported to be inhibitory for hepatoma cell growth. Some of these cytokines are therefore being used in clinical trials for patients with hepatoma, TNFα for example, but the results are rather controversial, as the preliminary response rates are unsatisfactory. In order to achieve a better response, larger doses (both systemic and regional) have been tested, but the wider use of cytokines is still hampered by the severe side effects suffered by patients: both general reactions from the foreign protein and the specific effects of the particular cytokine used (Creaven et al 1987, Niederle et al 1988, Wiedenmann et al 1989, van der Schelling et al 1992).

Other cytokines, on the other hand, stimulate hepatoma cell growth IL-1 and IL-6 have been shown to stimulate both hepatoma cell secretory functions (acute phase protein production) (Magielska-Zero et al 1988, Grunfeld et al 1991, Mackiewicz et al 1991, Ono et al 1992) and cell proliferation (Serve 1991). Other cytokines may only stimulate cancer cell growth, GM-CSF and IL-1 for example (Hamburger et al 1987). It is important to note that hepatoma cells themselves may also produce these stimulatory cytokines (Tohyama et al 1989, Northemann et al 1990, Tani et al 1990, Baffet et al 1991, Ross et al 1991) and therefore stimulate their growth by an autocrine mechanism. The administration of TNF or after liver resection (to surgically remove a hepatoma) may also induce IL-6 and IL-1 production and therefore in the treatment or recovery period a paracrine stimulation of growth of any residual hepatoma may occur.

Hepatoma cells, along with some other malignant cells, have been shown to be susceptible to treatment with fatty acids; a high level of toxicity to GLA and other fatty acids has been reported by several laboratories (Hayashi et al 1990, Horrobin 1990).

The relationship between cytokine and PUFA on the growth of malignant cells has been less well studied. Newman in 1990 reported that the inhibition of cancer cell growth induced by the cytokine TGFβ1 was polyunsaturated fatty acid dependent. This observation provokes fundamental questions about the requirements for PUFAs in the biological effects of cytokines on malignant cells.

We have examined the effects of PUFAs and a variety of cytokines separately and in combination on hepatoma cell growth.

Experimental methods

Cell line

The human hepatoma cell line PLC/PRF/5 (European Collections Of Animal Cell Culture, ECACC) was used and maintained in DMEM supplemented with 10% FCS, streptomycin, and penicillin.

Fatty acids and cytokines

GLA and linoleic acid (LA) were prepared in our standard way, as in the monocyte experiments. LiGLA, which is partially water soluble, was provided by Scotia Pharmaceutical Ltd, Guildford, England. Recombinant human cytokines IL-1β, IL-3, IL-4, IL-5, IL-6, IL-7, IL-10, TGFβ, TNFα, IFNγ, GM-CSF and HGF were stored in balanced salt solution with 1% BSA at −80°C as stock solutions; repeated thawing was avoided.

Cell growth assay

The well-established MTT method was used in this study as previously described. Briefly, cells suspended at 1×10^5/ml were plated onto 96-well tissue culture plates and allow to adhere to the floor for 4 h. The cytokines at various concentrations, or the different fatty acids (dissolved in ethanol at a final concentrations of less than 0.01%), or a combination, were then added to cells in triplicate. The plates were cultured for either 72 h in experiments to compare agents or from day 1 to day 6 in experiments to investigate the time course of the effect on cell growth. At the end of each culture period, MTT at a final concentration of 2.5 mg/ml was added to the cells and incubated for a further 4 h to allow the coloured crystals to develop. Triton X100, 10%, was added and left at 4°C overnight to solubilize the crystals. The absorbance was measured using a Titertek Multiscanner and cell growth was calculated as percentage growth compared with cells cultured in medium only. In selected cultures indomethacin, NDGA, tocopherol or a combination was also included to establish the possible contribution of fatty acids metabolites.

Morphology and DNA fragmentation of cells

At the end of the culture period the morphology of cells were observed both under phase contrast microscopy and after staining with crystal violet. In order to determine the existence of fragmented DNA (Cohen & Duke 1984), some cells were cultured with fatty acids, cytokines, or a combination of the two for 24 h, and then lysed with a buffer containing 20 mM EDTA, 0.5% Triton X100 and 5 mM Tris (pH 8.0) on ice. The fragmented DNA was then separated from intact DNA by ultracentrifugation at 27 000 **g**. The fragmented DNA content was then measured using Burton's diphenylamine method (Burton 1956).

Cytosolic free calcium and lipid content

Cytosolic free calcium was determined using dual wavelength fluorometry of fura-2 as described by Al-Mohanna & Hallett (1988). PLC/PRF/5 cells are loaded with fura-2 at room temperature and then the fluorescence corresponding to the resting level, after addition of fatty acid, or cytokines, or the combination of the two is recorded.

In order to observe the lipid content after culture the hepatoma cells were stained with oil red O-isopropyl alcohol solution and counterstained with methyl green.

Results

Regulation of hepatoma growth by fatty acids and cytokines

We confirm that hepatoma cells are sensitive to treatment with GLA and we have also shown that the cells show a similar response to its water soluble lithium salt (LiGLA) (Fig. 3.7). The effect is even more noticeable in the prolonged cultures. The cells are also sensitive to linoleic acid (LA) although this is not as pronounced as with GLA (data not shown).

In the presence of different cytokines, hepatoma cells showed different growth patterns; IL-4, IL-5, TGF-β, HGF, and IFNγ showed inhibitory effects on cell growth, while IL-1, IL-3, IL-10, IL-6, and GM-CSF showed stimulatory effects, TNFα however produces only a slight stimulation of growth (Table 3.3).

In order to determine whether fatty acids and cytokines have synergistic effects, combinations of cytokines and GLA or LiGLA were also tested. The sensitivity of the hepatoma cells to inhibitory cytokines was increased by GLA. Cells also became sensitive to TNFα in the presence of GLA and LiGLA. The stimulatory effects of IL-1, IL-3, IL-5, IL-6, IL-10 and

GM-CSF were reversed by both GLA and LiGLA (Table 3.3 and Figs 3.8, 3.9, 3.10).

Table 3.3. The effects of various cytokines on the growth of hepatoma cells as assayed by the MTT method

Cytokines	Cytokine only	Cytokine + GLA	Cytokine + LiGLA
IL-1β (25 U/ml)	110.4±5.6%	62.3±13.3%	90.6±0.3%
IL-3 (10 ng/ml)	119.2±4.9%	64.3±1.7%	91.7±1.0%
IL-4 (10 U/ml)	94.3±2.6%	64.1±5.7%	89.9±2.6%
IL-5 (10 ng/ml)	91.1±4.6%	59.5±1.1%	79.9±2.5%
IL-6 (250 U/ml)	111.9±6.5%	75.2±6.8%	90.8±1.2%
IL-7 (10 ng/ml)	92.8±4.0%	47.1±1.0%	72.6±1.1%
IL-10 (10 ng/ml)	106.5±2.5%	45.2±4.1%	70.1±0.3%
TGFβ (10 RU/ml)	85.3±2.1%	62.2±3.5%	70.0±1.2%
HGF (10 ng/ml)	91.2±0.9%	74.3±3.1%	87.2±3.2%
GM-CSF (10 ng/ml)	112.7±4.8%	88.5±5.5%	100.1±3%
TNFα (2 ng/ml)	104.8±5%	62.2±3.5%	93.6±2.6%
IFNγ (20 ng/ml)	94.6±2.9%	73.1±4.2%	83.7±0.9%

Cells were treated with cytokine only, cytokine plus GLA or LiGLA at 25 μM and were cultured for 72 h.

The effects were seen as early as culture day 1, and much larger effects were seen on day 3 (Fig. 3.8). There is a concentration-dependent effect with both GLA and cytokines and examples are shown in Fig. 3.9 and Fig. 3.10.

The possible contribution of FA metabolites

The possibility exists that the hepatoma may be sensitive to the metabolites of fatty acids. To test this hypothesis cyclooxygenase, lipoxygenase inhibitors, and an anti-oxidant, tocopherol were included in some of the cultures. The effects of fatty acids on hepatoma cells were not inhibited by NDGA or indomethacin (data not shown). Only tocopherol showed a slight inhibition on the effects of IL-6 with GLA, but both tocopherol alone or in combination with NDGA and indomethacin block only a part of the response (Fig. 3.11). The effects of other cytokines were not affected by any of the inhibitors. This suggests that the lipid peroxides may only partly contribute to the effects seen.

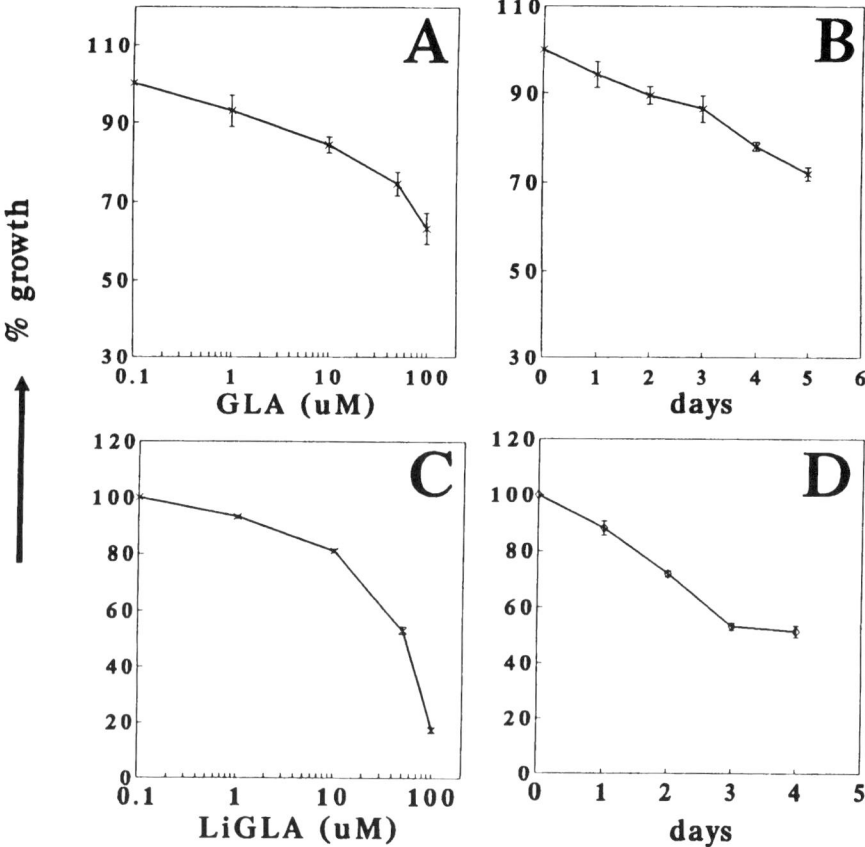

Fig. 3.7.   The sensitivity of PLC/PRF/5 hepatoma cells to the fatty acids, GLA, LiGLA. There is a dose-related effect on the cell growth (A and C) at 72 h. There is also a time-dependent effect with a constant fatty acid concentration (B and D).

Cytosolic free calcium and lipid content changes

No changes of cytosolic free calcium were seen with the addition of GLA (up to 200 μM), TNF (up to 10 ng/ml), TGFβ (up to 10 RU/ml), HGF (up to 40 ng/ml) or the combination of GLA and individual cytokines. We thank Dr M.B. Hallett for his help in measuring cytosolic free calcium.

With both phase contrast microscopy and oil red O stain there was a tremendously increased lipid content in the cells cultured with GLA and cytokines particularly with TNF and TGFβ.

Cell morphology and DNA fragmentation

At the end of the culture period, an assessment of cell morphology revealed that the majority of cells had undergone necrosis, but cells with

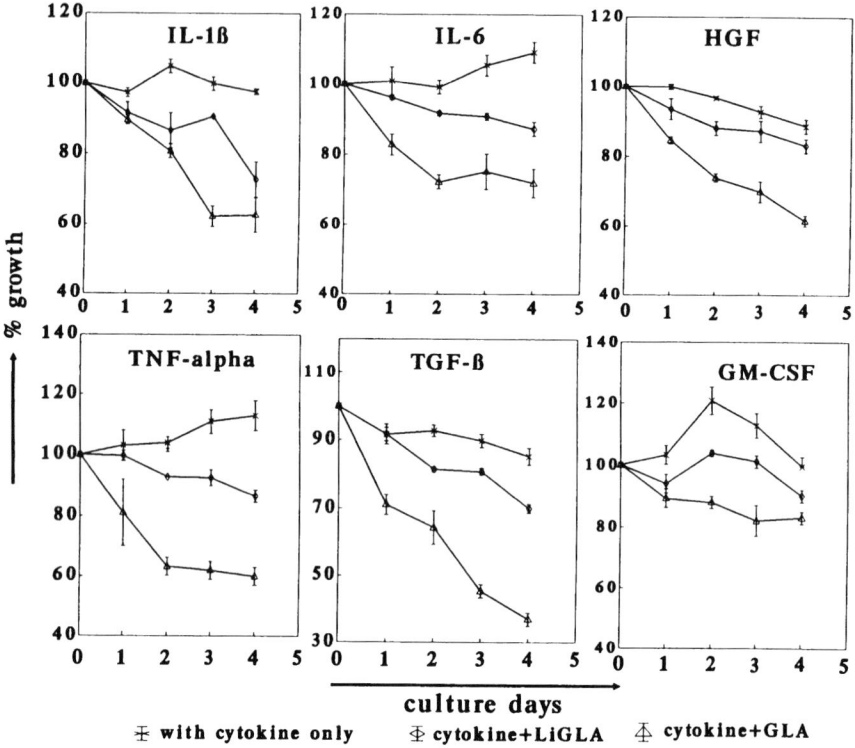

Fig. 3.8. The effects of GLA and LiGLA on cytokine induced hepatoma cell growth. In a 72 h culture GLA and LiGLA have an inhibitory effect with these cytokines used at the concentrations listed in Table 3.3.

condensed DNA (apoptosis) were also seen. A DPA assay revealed an increased content of fragmented DNA in the cells, particularly with the combination of GLA and cytokines (Fig 3.12) indicating that apoptosis is also a major event in this culture system.

OVERVIEW

It has been reported that GLA and other n-6 fatty acids possess anti-cancer properties; our data also show that GLA and its lithium salt inhibit hepatoma cell growth.

With the cytokines we have tested, cell sensitivity is variable. Though HGF has initially been shown to stimulate normal hepatocyte DNA synthesis (Matsumoto et al 1991), our data, together with the most recent work from Shiota et al (1992), suggest that HGF inhibits hepatoma cell growth which is in clear distinction to normal hepatocytes. IFNγ and TGFβ also show an inhibitory effect on hepatoma cell growth which is in keeping with others' reports. IL-1β, IL-3, IL-10, IL-6 and GM-CSF how-

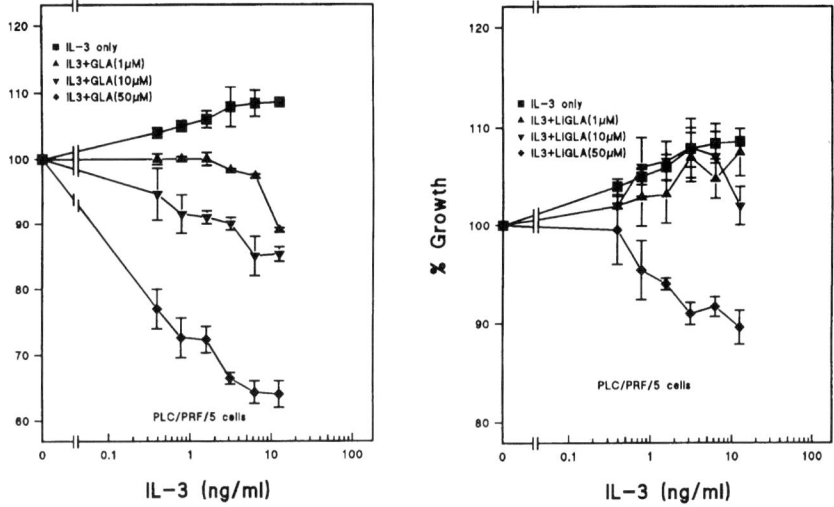

Fig. 3.9. Concentration depdendent effect of both GLA and LiGLA on IL-3 induced PLC/PRF/5 cell growth. The stimulatory effects of IL-3 are reversed and an inhibitory effect was seen with the presence of GLA as low as 1 μM.

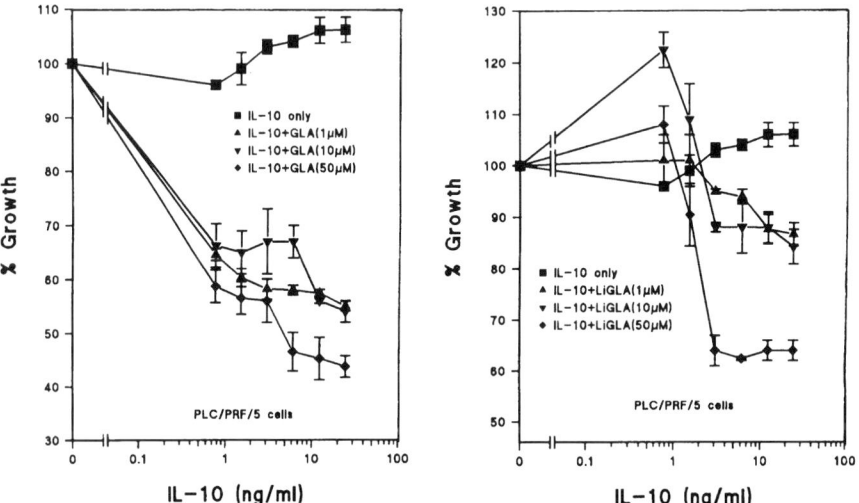

Fig. 3.10. Concentration dependent effects of both GLA and LiGLA on IL-10 induced PLC/PRF/5 cell growth. The stimulatory effects of IL-10 are reversed and an inhibitory effect was seen with the presence of GLA as low as 1 μM. Very low concentrations of IL-10 however appear to cause increased stimulation with LiGLA.

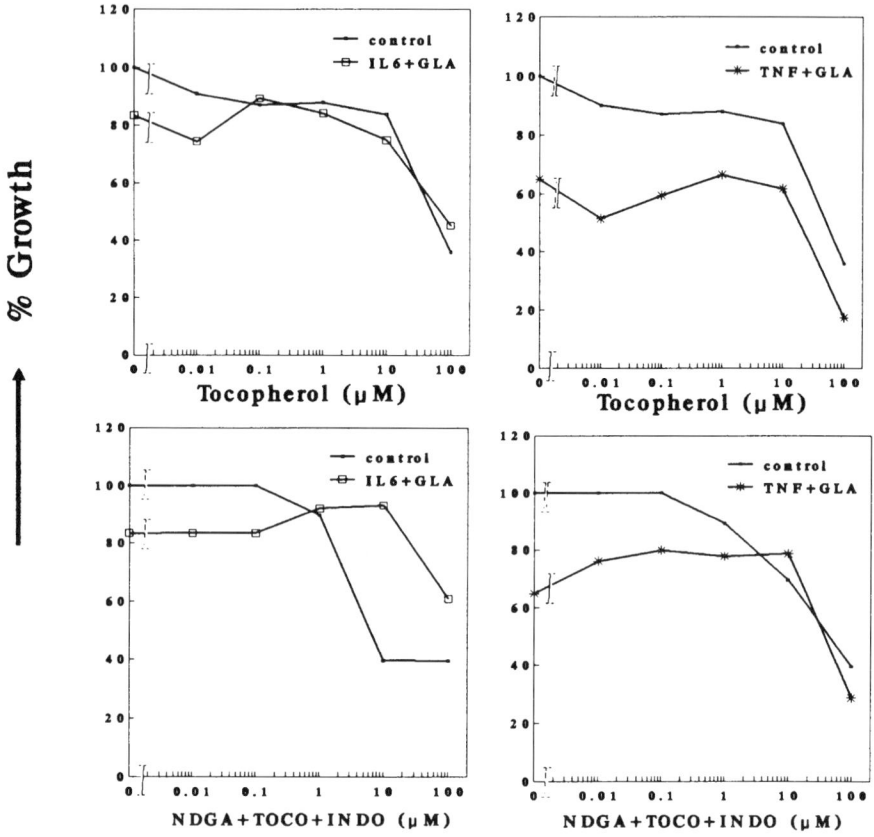

Fig. 3.11. Fatty acids metabolites and cytokine induced hepatoma growth. Cells were cultured with GLA or LiGLA plus cytokine and tocopherol alone or in combination with NDGA, and indomethacin for 72 h. The IL-6 and GLA induced cell growth inhibition was partly blocked by tocopherol. Whereas TNF or TNF and GLA combination were not affected as was the case with all the other cytokine and cytokine with GLA combinations tested.

ever show a stimulatory effect. Although it has been previously reported that TNF might inhibit proliferation of some cells our data show that the growth of PLC/PRF/5 cells is up-regulated as has been reported by many others (Balkwill 1993). In common with gastric carcinoma (Morisaki et al 1992), hepatoma cell growth is also inhibited by IL-4.

The data presented here also clearly demonstrates that the polyunsaturated fatty acid GLA is essential in cytokine-mediated hepatoma cell growth inhibition. As reported by Newman, the inhibitory effects of TGFβ1 are greatly enhanced by GLA and LiGLA, and the effects of HGF and IFNγ are also markedly increased. The other interesting observation is that the growth stimulation of the stimulatory cytokines, namely, IL-1β, IL-3, IL-6, IL-10 and GM-CSF are reversed by these fatty acids. The

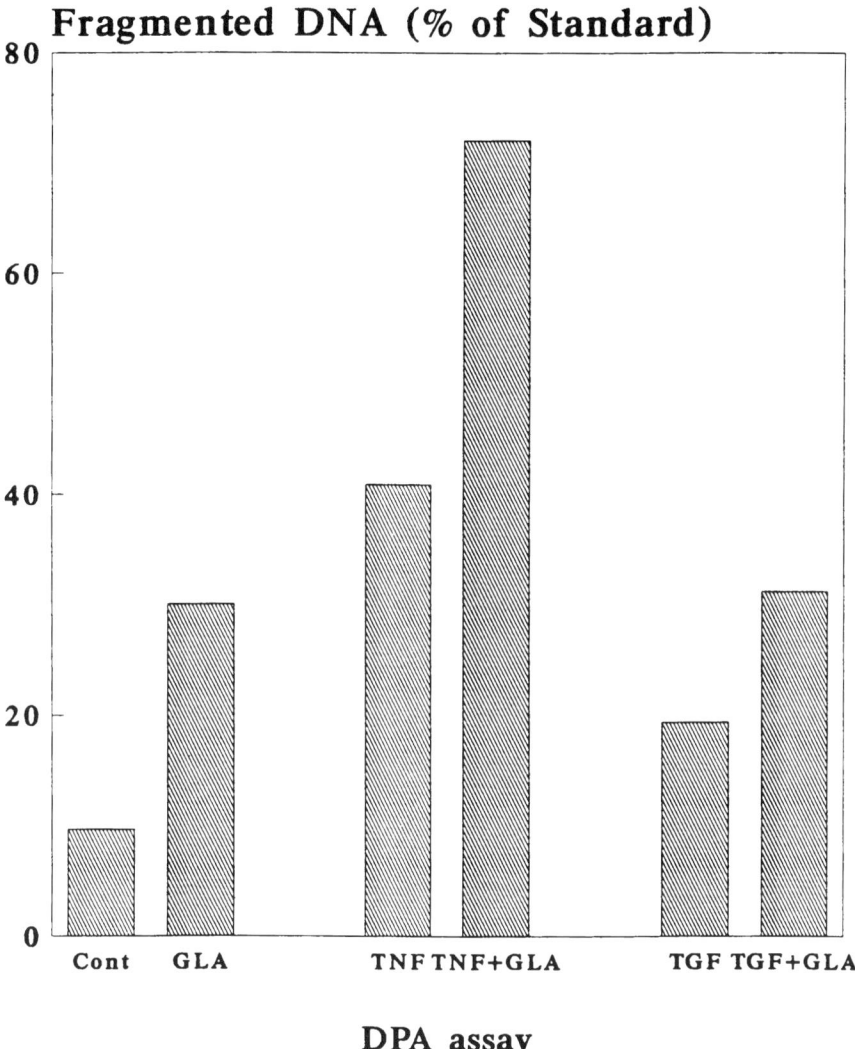

Fig. 3.12.   DNA fragmentation of hepatoma cells. Cells were cultured with fatty acid alone or together with cytokine for 24 h. Cells were then lysed and fragmented DNA was separated from intact DNA by ultracentrifugation. The content of fragmented DNA was measured by the DPA method. GLA alone or in combination with TNFα and TGFβ induced a high proportion of DNA fragmentation. GLA cultures are significantly greater than non-GLA cultures. Cytokine plus GLA cultures are significantly greater than cytokine only cultures. Student's *t*-test, *P*<0.01 taken as significant.

cells which are not sensitive to TNF alone show sensitivity to TNF in the presence of GLA and LiGLA.

The synergistic inhibition of hepatoma growth by GLA and cytokines may be of clinical interest. The clinical trials using TNFα, and other cytokines are unsatisfactory, either because of intolerable side effects, or because of tumour insensitivity or even increased cell growth and motility with TNF (Balkwill 1993). There is also a concern with the use of GM-CSF and IL-3 as adjuvant agents in chemotherapy (Kurzrock et al 1991, Schulz et al 1991, Orazi et al 1992) as they may stimulate cancer cell growth (Foulke et al 1990, Nachbaur et al 1990, Dippold & zem Buschenfelde 1991). Our data confirms this point. While the combination of cytokines fails to improve the response rate (Schiller et al 1992), the combination of fatty acids like GLA or more practically LiGLA with cytokines may increase the cell sensitivity to a variety of cytokines and at the same time reverse the unwanted effects of other cytokines, GM-CSF for example.

The other potential use for GLAs in this area is with patients who receive operations. Nakazaki (1992) described an important finding that after resection of a hepatoma there is a significant and sustained elevation of blood IL-1α and β, IL-6, TNF, and GM-CSF. For those patients with recurrence after surgery, the levels of IL-1 and TNF are rather higher than in the case of non-recurrence. The phenomenon is also seen with other gastrointestinal cancers after surgery. The author suggests that the postoperative increases in the levels of these cytokines may be responsible for the recurrence. Similar cytokine changes have also been reported in patients undergoing IL-2 and TNF treatment for cancer (van Haelst Pisani et al 1991). IL-1 and other cytokines (Arguello et al 1992) are known to be stimulatory for cancer metastases. Our data described here may provide some evidence that IL-1, IL-3, IL-6, TNF, and GM-CSF are also stimulatory for hepatoma growth. The use of GLA for these patients may help to overcome the problems observed after liver resection.

The precise mechanisms of the anticancer properties of essential fatty acids are not clear. Horrobin and colleagues (1990) has suggested that lipid peroxidation may contribute to the mechanism. Our data shows that only some of the effects are due to this mechanism; the effects of IL-6 and GLA in combination is reversed by tocopherol. It is established that PUFA supplementation in vitro may be incoporated into plasma cell membrane quickly and then modify membrane function and hence cell functions. This is a possible mechanism for GLA-induced cytokine effects in these cells. It worth noting that PUFA may also modify the nuclear lipid composition (Chapkin et al 1992), where with the supplementation of both n-6 and n-3 fatty acids n-3 PUFA are retained and sn-2 18:2 n-6 is sacrificed. These changes may regulate gene functions and intranuclear signal exchanges. The relationship between this and DNA fragmentation remain to be elucidated.

Although there are reports indicating that PUFAs may induce cytosolic free calcium changes, this does not seem to be the mechanism where GLA or GLA and cytokine exert their effects here as none of the treatments induced cytosolic free calcium changes as measured in our study.

It has recently been shown that PUFA may induce genetic changes and also that tumour cells at different phases have different PUFA levels (Pan et al 1990). GLA may also induce some of these changes, and more work is needed in this area.

We conclude that the n-6 fatty acid GLA alone, at low concentrations, inhibits cell growth and synergistically increases the growth inhibition of the PLC/PRF/5 hepatoma cells induced by IFNγ, TGFβ, and HGF. GLA increases the sensitivity of the cells to TNFα, but reverses the stimulatory effects of GM-CSF, IL-1, IL-3 and IL-6. The effects seem only partially due to lipid peroxidation as tocopherol only partly blocks the effects, while indomethacin, and NDGA have no influence on the GLA effect. This suggests that there may be a place for the use of fatty acids in some cancer patients, particularly in combination with cytokines, as the potential importance of cytokines in cancer treatment is becoming recognized (Greiner 1991), and many current clinical trials using cytokines in cancer patients are unsatisfactory.

ABBREVIATIONS

AA: arachidonic acid;
ARDS: adult respiratory distress syndrome;
BSA: bovine serum albumin;
DPA: diphenylamine;
EFA: essential fatty acids;
FCS: fetal calf serum;
GLA: gamma-linolenic acid;
GM-CSF: granulocyte-macrophage colony-stimulating factor;
HEX: hexosaminidase;
HGF/SF: hepatocyte growth factor/scatter factor;
IFN: interferon;
INDO: indomethacin;
LA: linoleic acid;
LPS: lipopolysaccheraide;
LiGLA: GLA lithium salt;
IL,1,2,3,4,5,6,7,8,10,11,12: interleukin-1,2,3,4,5,6,7,8,10,11,12;
MNC: mononuclear cells;
MTT: 3-[4,5-dimethylthiazol-2-yl]-2.5-diphenyltetrazolium bromide;
NDGA: nordihydroguaiaretic acid;
NSE: non-specific esterase;
PG: prostaglandin;
PUFA: polyunsaturated fatty acids;
TGFβ: transforming growth factor beta;
TNFα: tumour necrosis factor alpha;
TOCO: tocopherol.

REFERENCES

Al-Mohanna FA, Hallett MB 1988 The use of fura-2 to determine the relationship between cytoplasmic free Ca^{2+} and oxidase activation in rat neutrophils. Cell Calcium 9: 17–26
Arguello F, Baggs RB, Graves BT, Harwell SE, Cohen HJ, Frantz CN 1992 Effect of IL-1 on experimental bone/bone-marrow metastases. International Journal of Cancer 52: 802–807

Baffet G, Braciak TA, Fletcher RG, Gauldie J, Fey GH, Northmann W 1991 Autocrine activity of interleukin-6 secreted by hepatocarcinoma cell lines. Molecular Biology and Medicine 8: 141–156

Balkwill F 1993 Tumour necrosis factor: improving on the formula. Nature 361: 206–207

Bartoli GM, Bartoli S, Galiotti T, Bertoli E 1980 Superoxide dismutase content and microsomal lipid composition of tumors with different growth rates. Biochimica et Biophysica Acta 620: 205–211

Belch JJF, Ansell D, Madhok R, O'Dowd A, Sturrock RD 1988 Effects of altering dietary essential fatty acids on requirements for non-steroidal anti-inflammatory drugs in patients with rheumatoid arthritis: a double-blind placebo controlled study. Annals of the Rheumatic Diseases. 47: 96–104

Bemelmans MHA, Gouma DJ, Greve JW, Buurman WA 1992 Cytokines tumor-necrosis factor and interleukin-6 in experimental biliary obstruction in mice. Hepatology 15: 1132–1136

Beyaert R, Fiers W 1992 Potentiation of tumour necrosis factor-mediated activities by lithium salts: a review. Lithium 3: 181–189

Blamey SL, Fearon KCH, Gilmour WH, Osborne DH, Carter DC 1983 Prediction of risk in biliary surgery. British Journal of Surgery 70: 535–538

Burton K 1956 A study of the conditions and mechanism of the diphenylamine reaction for the colorimetric estimation of deoxyribonucleic acid. Biochemical Journal 62: 315–323

Chapkin RS, Davidson LD, Davidson LA 1992 Phospholipid molecular species composition of mouse liver nuclei. Biochemical Journal 287: 237–240

Chatterjee SK, Chowjury K, Bhattacharya M, Barlow JJ 1982 Beta-hexosaminidase activities and isozymes in normal ovary and ovarian adenocarcinoma. Cancer 49: 128–135

Cheeseman KH, Collins M, Proudfoot K, Slater TF, Burton GW, Webb AC, Ingold KV 1986 Studies in lipid peroxidation in normal and tumor tissues. Biochemical Journal 235: 507–514

Cohen JJ, Duke RC 1984 Glucocorticoid activation of a calcium dependent endonuclease in thymocyte nuclei leads to cell death. Journal of Immunology. 132: 38–42

Creaven PJ, Plager JE, Dupere S 1987 Phase I clinical trial of recombinant human tumor necrosis factor. Cancer Chemotherapy and Pharmacology 20: 137–144

Das UN, Begin ME, Ells G, Huang YS, Horrobin DF 1987 Polyunsaturated fatty acids augment free radical generation in tumor cells in vitro. Biochemical Biophysical Research Communications 145: 15–24

Das UN 1990 Gamma-linolenic acid, arachidonic acid, and eicosapentaenoic acid as potential anticancer drugs. Nutrition 6: 429–434

Dippold W, zem Buschenfelde KM 1991 Proliferation of gastrointestinal carcinoma cells by T lymphocyte factors interleukin-3 and granulocyte–macrophage colony-stimulating factor. Immunologic Research 10: 258–260

Dunbar LM, Bailey JM 1975 Enzyme deletions and essential fatty acid metabolism in cultured cells. Journal of Biological Chemistry 250: 1152–1153

Eskandari MK, Bolgos G, Miller C, Nguyen DT, DeForge LE, Remick DG 1992 Anti-tumor necrosis factor antibody therapy fails to prevent lethality after cecal ligation and puncture or endotoxemia. Journal of Immunology 148: 2724–2730

Fischer E, Marano MA, Wan Zee KJ, Rock CS, Hawes AS, Thompson WA, DeForge L, Kenney JS, Remick DG, Bloedow DC, Thompson RC, Lowry SF, Moldawer LL 1992 Interleukin-1 receptor blockage improve survival and hemodynamic performance in *Escherichia coli* septic shock, but fails to alter host responses to sublethal endotoxemia. Journal of Clinical Investigation 89: 1551–1557

Fong Y, Tracey KJ, Moldawer LL, Hesse DG, Manogue KB, Kenney JS, Lee AT, Kuo GC, Allison AC, Lowry SF, Cerami A 1989 Antibodies to cachectin/tumor necrosis factor reduce interleukin-1β and interleukin-6 appearance during lethal bacteremia. Journal of Experimental Medicine 170: 1627–1633

Foulke RS, Martha MH, Trotta PP, von Hoff DD 1990 In vitro assessment of the effects of granulocyte–macrophage colony-stimulating factor on primary human tumors and derived lines. Cancer Research 50: 6264–6267

Greiner JW, Smalley RV, Borden EC, Martin EW, Guadagni F, Roselli M, Schlom J 1991 Application of monoclonal antibodies and recombinant cytokines for the treatment of human colorectal and other carcinomas. Journal of Surgical Oncology Supplement 2: 9–13

Grunfeld C, Dinarello CA, Feingold KR 1911 Tumor necrosis factor-α, interleukin-1 and interferon alpha stimulate triglyceride synthesis in HEP G2 cells. Metabolism 40: 894–898

Hagve TA 1988 Effects of unsaturated fatty acids on cell membrane functions. Scandinavian Journal of Clinical Investigation 48: 381–388

Hamburger AW, Lurie KA, Condon ME 1987 Stimulation of anchorage-independent growth of human tumor cells by interleukin-1. Cancer Research 47: 5612–5615

Hayashi Y, Fukushima S, Hirata T, Kishimoto S, Katsuki T, Nakano M 1990 Anti-cancer activity of free γ-linolenic acid on AH-109A rat hepatoma cells and the effect of serum albumin on the anti-cancer activity of γ-linolenic acid in vitro. Journal of Pharmacobio-Dynamics 13: 705–711

Holman JM, Rikkers LF, Moody FG 1979 Sepsis in the management of complicated biliary disorders. American Journal of Surgery 138: 809–813

Holman JM, Rikkers LF 1982 Biliary obstruction and host defense failure. Journal of Surgical Research 32: 208–213

Horrobin DF 1990 Essential fatty acids, lipid peroxidation, and cancer. In: Horrobin Omega-6 essential fatty acids. Pathophysiology and roles in clinical medicine. Wiley–Liss, New York, pp 351–379

Hunt DR, Allison MEM, Prentice CRM, Blumgart LH 1982 Endotoxemia disturbance of coagulation and obstructive jaundice. American Journal of Surgery 144: 325–329

Hwang D 1989 Essential fatty acids and immune responses. FASEB Journal 3: 2052–2061

Jiang WG, Puntis MCA, Hughes LE 1991 Monocyte lysosomal enzyme secretion in jaundice. European Surgical Research 23: Supplement 1, 110

Jiang WG, Puntis MCA, Hallett MB 1992 Neutrophil oxidative response and its relationship to clinical outcome in jaundiced patients. HPB Surgery, Supplement, 104.

Kleinerman ES, Knowles RD, Blick MB, Zwelling LA 1989 Lithium chloride stimulates human monocytes to secrete tumor necrosis factor/cachectin. Journal of Leukocyte Biology 46: 484–492

Kunkel SL, Ogawa H, Ward PA 1981 Suppression of chronic inflammation by evening primrose oil. Progress in Lipid Research 20: 885–889

Kurzrock R, Talpaz M, Estov Z, Rosenblum MG, Gutterman JV 1991 Phase I study of recombinant human interleukin-3 in patients with bone marrow failure. Journal of Clinical Oncology 9: 1241–1250

Lokesh BR, Wrann M 1984 Incorporation of palmitic acid or oleic acid into macrophage membrane lipids exerts differential effects on the function of normal mouse peritoneal macrophages. Biochimica et Biophysica Acta 792: 141–148

Mackiewicz A, Speroff T, Ganapathi MK, Kushner I 1991 Effects of cytokine combinations on acute phase protein production in two human hepatoma cell lines. Journal of Immunology 146: 3032–3037

Magielska-Zero D, Bereta J, Czuba-Pelech B, Pajdak W, Gauldie J, Koi A 1988 Inhibitory effect of human recombinant interferon gamma on synthesis of acute phase protein in human hepatoma Hep-G2 cells stimulated by leukocyte cytokines, TNF alpha and IFN-beta 2/BSF-2/IL-6. Biochemistry International 17: 17–23

Matsumoto K, Tajima H, Nakamura T 1991 Hepatocyte growth factor is a potent stimulator of human melanocyte DNA synthesis and growth. Biochemical and Biophysical Research Communication 176: 45–51

Mohoney EM, Scott WA, Landsberger FR, Hamill AL, Cohn ZA 1980 Influence of fatty acyl substitute on the composition and function of macrophage membrane. Journal of Biological Chemistry 255: 4910–4917

Morisaki T, Yuzuki DH, Lin RT, Foshag LT, Morton DL, Hoon DSB 1992 Interleukin-4 receptor expression and growth inhibition of gastric carcinoma cells by interleukin-4. Cancer Research 52: 6059–6065

Mozes T, Ben-Efraim S, Tak CJAM, Heiligers JPC, Saxena P R, Bonta I L 1991 Serum levels of tumor necrosis factor determine fatal or non-fatal course of endotoxic shock. Immunology Letters 1991 27: 157–162

Nachbaur D, Denz H, Zwiezina H, Schmalzl F, Huber H 1990 Stimulation of colony formation of various human carcinoma cell lines by rhGM-CSF and rhIL-3. Cancer Letters 50: 197–201

Nakazaki H 1992 Preoperative and postoperative cytokines in patients with cancer. Cancer 70: 709–713

Neale ML, Williams BD, Matthews N 1989 Tumour necrosis factor activity in joint fluids from rheumatoid patients. British Journal of Rheumatology 28: 104–108

Newman MJ 1990 Inhibition of carcinoma and melanoma cell growth by type 1 transforming growth factor β is dependent on the presence of polyunsaturated fatty acids. Proceedings of the National Academy of Science of USA 87: 5543–5547

Niederle N, Moritz T, Kurschel E 1988 Recombinant human tumor necrosis factor alpha (TNF) in the treatment of advanced malignancies: a phase I study. Proceedings of American Association of Cancer Research 29: 431

Northemann W, Hattori M, Baffet G, Braciak TA, Fletcher RG, Abraham IJ, Gauldie J, Baumann M, Fey GH 1990 Production of interleukin-6 by hepatoma cells. Molecular Biology and Medicine 7: 273–285

Ono M, Kohda H, Kawaguchi T, Ohhira M, Sekiya C, Namiki M, Takeyasu A, Taniguchi N 1992 Induction of Mn-superoxide dismutase by tumor necrosis factor, interleukin-1 and interleukin-6 in human hepatoma cells. Biochemical Biophysical Research Communications 182: 1100–1107

Opal SM, Cross AS, Sadoff JC, Collins HH, Kelly NM, Victor GH, Palardy JE, Bodmer MW 1991 Efficacy of antilipopolysaccharide and anti-tumor necrosis factor monoclonal antibodies in a neutropenic rat model of pseudomonas sepsis. Journal of Clinical Investigation 88: 885–890

Orazi A, Catteretti G, Schiro R, Siena S, Bregni M, Di Nicola M, Gianni AM 1992 Recombinant human interleukin-3 and granulocyte–macrophage colony-stimulating factor administration in vivo after high dose cyclophosphamide cancer therapy: effect on hematopoitic and microenvironment in human bone marrow. Blood 79: 2610–2619

O'Riodain MG, Collins KH, Pilz M, Saporoschetz IB, Mannick JA, Rodrick ML 1992 Modulation of macrophage-hyperactivity improves survival in a burn-sepsis model. Archives of Surgery 127: 152–158

Pain JA, Cahill CJ, Bailey ME, 1985 Perioperative complications in obstructive jaundice: therapeutic considerations. British Journal of Surgery 72: 942–945

Pain JA 1987 Reticuloendothelial function in obstructive jaundice. British Journal of Surgery 74: 1091–1094

Pan DA, Sullivan-Tailyour G, Hulbert AJ 1990 Membrane fatty acid changes during the cell cycle of CV-1 cells. Experimental Cell Research 191: 141–143

Puntis MCA, Jiang WG 1991 Neutrophil increase their respiratory burst but fail to be primed by TNF in obstructive jaundice. Journal Leukocyte Biology Suppl 2: 78

Puntis MCA, Jiang WG 1992a Monocytes from obstructive jaundice patients show increased TNF and IL-6 production. British Journal of Surgery 79: 458–459

Puntis MCA, Jiang WG 1992b Increased monocyte TNF production in malignant jaundice and its relation to prognosis. European Journal of Surgical Oncology, in press

Redmond HP, Chavin KD, Bromberg JS, Daly JM 1991 Inhibition of macrophage-activating cytokines is beneficial in the acute septic response. Annals of Surgery 214: 502–509

Reid T, Chakkodabylu SR, Ringold GM 1991 Resistance to killing by tumour necrosis factor in an adipocyte cell line caused by a defect in arachidonic acid biosythesis. Journal of Biological Chemistry 266: 16580–16586

Renz H, Gong JH, Schmidt A, Nain M, Gemsa D 1988 Release of tumor necrosis factor-alpha from macrophages: enhancement and suppression are dose-dependently regulated by prostaglandin E_2 and cyclic nucleotides. Journal of Immunology. 141: 2388–2393

Rosenthal AS, Shevach EM 1973 Function of macrophages in antigen recognition by guinea pig T lymphocytes. I. Requirement for histocompatible macrophages and lymphocytes. Journal of Experimental Medicine 135: 1194–1212

Ross HJ, Sato N, Ueyama Y, Koeffler HP 1991 Cytokine messenger RNA stability is enhanced in tumor cells. Blood 77: 1787–1795

Sakai T, Yamaguchi T, Shiroko Y, Sekiguchi M, Fujii G, Nishino H 1984 Prostaglandin D_2 inhibits the proliferation of human malignant tumor cells. Prostaglandins 27: 17–26

Schiller JH, Witt PL, Storer B, Alberti D, Tombes MB, Arzoomanian R, Brown RR, Proctor RA, Voss SD, Spriggs DS, Trump DL, Borden EC 1992 Clinical and biologic effects of combination therapy with gamma-interferon and tumor necrosis factor. Cancer 69: 562–571

Schroit AJ, Gallily R 1979 Macrophage fatty acid composition and phagocytosis. Effect of unsaturation on cellular phagocytic activity. Immunology, 36: 199–205

Schulz G, Krumwieh D, Oster W, 1991, Adjuvant therapy with recombinant interleukin-3 and granulocyte–macrophage colony-stimulating factor. Pharmacology and Therapeutics 52: 85–94.

Scriven M W, Stewart J C W, Horrobin D F, Puntis M C A 1992. The pattern of plasma cholesterol ester fatty acids is abnormal in obstructive jaundice. HPB Surgery 5: supplement, 32

Serve H, Steinhauser G, Oberberg D, Flegel W A, Northoff H, Berdel W E 1991 Studies on the interaction between interleukin-6 and human malignant non-hematopoietic cell lines. Cancer Research 51: 3862–3866

Shevach E M, Tosenthal A S 1973 Function of macrophages in antigen recognition by guinea pig T lymphocytes. II. Role of macrophage in the regulation of genetic control of the immune responses. Journal of Experimental Medicine 138: 1213–1229

Shiota G, Rhoads D B, Wang TC, Nakamura T, Schmidt E 1992 Hepatocyte growth factor inhibits growth of hepatocellular carcinoma cells. Proceedings of the National Academy of Science of USA 89: 373–377

Socher S H, Martinez D, Craig J B, Kyhn J G, Oliff A 1988 Tumor necrosis factor not detectable in patients with clinical cancer cachexia. Journal of the National Cancer Institute 80: 2069–2073

Starnes H F, Pearce M K, Tewari A, Yim J H, Zou J C, Abams J S 1990 Anti-IL-6 monoclonal antibodies protect against lethal *Escherichia coli* infection and lethal tumor necrosis factor-alpha challenge in mice. Journal of Immunology 149: 4185–4191

Tanaka H, Ogura H, Yokota J, Sugimoto H, Yoshioka T, Sugimoto T 1991 Acceleration of superoxide production from leukocytes in trauma patients. Annals of Surgery 214: 187–192

Tani K, Ozawa K, Ogura H, Shimane M, Shirafuji N, Tsurota T, Yokota J, Nagata S, Ueyama Y, Takaku F 1990 Expression of granulocyte and granulocyte–macrophage colony-stimulating factors by human non-hematopoietic tumor cells. Growth Factors 3: 325–331

Tohyama K, Yoshida Y, Kubo A, Sudo T, Moriyama M, Sato H, Uchino H 1989 Detection of granulocyte-stimulating factor produced by a newly established human hepatoma cell line using a simple bioassay system. Japanese Journal of Cancer Research 80: 335–340

Trautinger F, Hammerle A F, Poschl G, Micksche M 1991 Respiratory burst capability of polymorphonuclear neutrophils and TNF-alpha serum levels in relationship to the development of septic syndrome in critically ill patients. Journal of Leukocyte Biology 49: 449–454

Trigger D R 1990 Essential fatty acids in primary biliary cirrhosis. In: Horrobin DF (ed) Omega-6 essential fatty acids. Pathophysiology and roles in clinical medicine. Wiley-Liss, New York pp 437–446

Tsao D, Freeman H J, Kim Y S 1979 β-hexosaminidase isozymes in tissue, cultured cells and media from human fetal intestine and colonic adenocarcinoma. Cancer Research 39: 3405–3410

van der Schelling G P, Ijzermans J N M, Kok T C, Scheringa M, Marquet R L, Splinter T A W, Jeekel J 1992 A phase I study of local treatment of liver metastasis with recombinant tumour necrosis factor. European Journal of Cancer. 28: 1073–1078

van Haelst Pisani C, Kovach J S, Kita H, Leiferman K M, Gleich G J, Silver J E, Dennin R, Abrams J S 1991 Administration of interleukin-2 (IL-2) results in increased plasma concentration of IL-5 and eosinophilia in patients with cancer. Blood 78: 1538–1544

Wait R B, Kahng K V 1989 Renal failure complicating obstructive jaundice. American Journal of Surgery. 157: 256–263

Wardle E N, Wright N A 1970 Endotoxin and acute renal failure associated with obstructive jaundice. British Medical Journal 4: 472–474

Wiedenmann B, Reichardt P, Rath U et al 1989 Phase I trial of intravenous continuous infusion of tumor necrosis factor in advanced metastatic carcinomas. Journal of Cancer Research and Clinical Oncology 115: 189–192

Yang-Yi Fan, Chapkin RS 1992 Mouse peritoneal macrophage prostaglandin E_1 synthesis is altered by dietary gamma-linolenic acid. Journal of Nutrition 122: 1600–1606

Zielinski CC, Mueller C, Tyl E, Tichatschek E, Kubista E, Spona J 1990 Impaired production of tumor necrosis factor in breast cancer. Cancer 66: 1944–1948

Ziegler EJ, Fisher CJ, Sprung CL, Straube RC et al 1991 Treatment of Gram-negative bacteremia and septic shock with HA-1A human monoclonal antibody against endotoxin. New England Journal of Medicine 324: 429–436

4. A phase II study of gamma-linolenic acid in pancreatic cancer and its effects on immune function and cytokine production

J. S. Falconer   J. A. Ross   K. C. H. Fearon

INTRODUCTION

Pancreatic cancer is now the fifth commonest cause of cancer death in the Western world (Williamson 1988). Despite recent improvements in diagnosis and staging, the prognosis remains poor with a median survival of approximately 3–6 months (Cancer of the Pancreas Task Force Group 1981, Williamson 1988). Surgical resection of early disease offers the only chance of long-term survival but is rarely feasible since most patients present with advanced disease (Carter 1989). Pancreatic cancer is also associated with substantial morbidity. For example, patients have a very high incidence of cachexia (De Wys 1986), and indeed, progressive weight loss is often the major symptom experienced. Clearly the best way to reverse such cachexia is to provide effective treatment of the cancer (Calman 1982). However, at present there is no effective systemic antineoplastic therapy for advanced pancreatic cancer (Carter 1989) and the toxicity of conventional chemotherapy may contribute further to the deteriorating nutritional status of the patient. Hence there is an urgent need for new selective (and therefore non-toxic) approaches to the management of patients with advanced pancreatic malignancy.

A number of studies have suggested that certain polyunsaturated fatty acids (PUFAs) such as eicosapentaenoic acid (EPA) and gamma-linolenic acid (GLA) can inhibit the growth of a variety of human cancer cell lines in vitro (Wica et al 1979, Dippenaar et al 1982, Fugiwara et al 1983, Begin et al 1985, 1986). Moreover, the effects of PUFAs have been shown to be selective for cancer cells without affecting normal cells in vitro (Begin et al 1986). It has also been shown that diets supplemented with the PUFAs EPA and GLA inhibit tumour growth in a variety of tumour-bearing mouse models (Karmali et al 1984, 1987, Pritchard et al 1989, Beck et al 1991). However, there is no information on the effects of such fatty acids in human pancreatic cancer.

In order to test the potential of PUFAs for the treatment of patients with pancreatic cancer, we have examined the effects of a variety of fatty acids on the growth in vitro of human pancreatic cancer cell lines.

The effects of these fatty acids on the growth of the three human pancreatic cancer cell lines MIA PaCa-2, PANC-1 and CFPAC over a 7 d culture period are summarised in Fig. 4.1. Both the polyunsaturated fatty acids EPA and GLA had a marked inhibitory effect on the growth of all three human pancreatic cancer cell lines at concentrations which might be achievable in vivo. In contrast, the saturated fatty acid stearic acid and mono-saturate oleic acid had no such effect.

With the knowledge that, at least in vitro, GLA could dramatically inhibit the growth of human pancreatic cancer cells, we have undertaken a phase II clinical trial of GLA in pancreatic cancer. GLA was a particularly interesting agent to use because not only might it have direct anti-tumour effects but, in theory, could improve some of the metabolic and immunological changes that are thought to contribute to cancer cachexia.

It is well known that tumour progression is associated with the development of both immunosuppression (Monson et al 1986) and marked

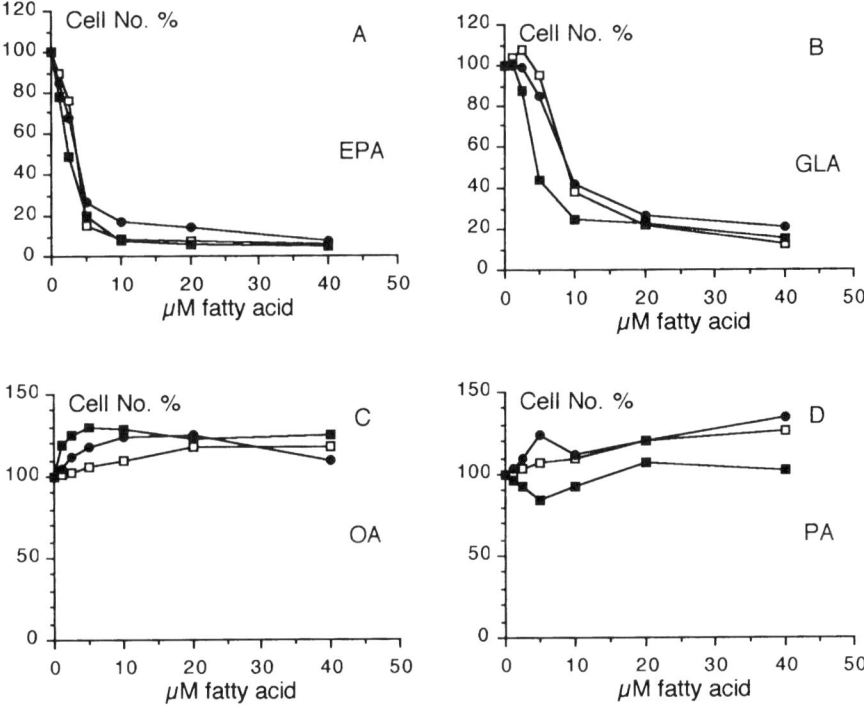

Fig. 4.1 Effect of increasing concentrations of the fatty acids (A) eicosapentaenoic acid (EPA), (B) gamma-linolenic acid (GLA), (C) oleic acid (OA) and (D) palmitic acid (PA) on the growth of the three human pancreatic cancer cell lines MIA PaCa-2(□), PANC-1(●) and CFPAC (■) over a 7-d period. Cell numbers are expressed as % control (without fatty acid). Each point represents the mean of at least three separate experiments.

cachexia. Such cachexia may be due to increased host production of potentially catabolic cytokines such as IL-6 and TNF (Fearon 1992). Moreover there is a potential link between T-cell function and enhanced cytokine production in cancer patients (Gough et al 1992). Recently we have confirmed that pancreatic cancer patients have impaired T-cell function and increased peripheral blood mononuclear cell (PBMC) tumour necrosis factor (TNF) production (Table 4.1) when compared with age- and sex-matched controls. However a cause and effect relationship between impaired T-cell function and abnormal cytokine release has still to be established.

PUFAs such as GLA and EPA have been shown to improve T-cell function (Calmus et al 1985, Cerra et al 1990) and down-regulate cytokine production (Endres et al 1989) in vivo. However, it is not known what effect such fatty acid manipulation might have on these parameters in cancer patients. Nor is it known what effect such manipulation might have on the development of cancer cachexia.

Table 4.1   T-cell function (phytohaemagglutinin (PHA)-stimulated PBMC [^{3}H]-thymidine uptake) and cytokine production (spontaneous PBMC TNF production) by healthy controls ($n =10$) and pancreatic cancer patients ($n =8$) (mean ± SEM)

	Control	Cancer
Thymidine uptake (counts/min/10^5 cells)	11239 ± 1045	9417 ± 1467*
TNF production (pg/ml/10^5 cells)	192 ± 48	804 ± 198*

*$P<0.01$, Student's t-test.

PATIENTS AND METHODS

Study protocol

Patients ($n =18$) received a 10 d, continuous infusion of GLA as its lithium salt. The dose was increased over the first 5 d and then continued at the maximum tolerated dose for the subsequent 5 d. The aim was to achieve a maximum dose of 10 g/d of GLA for this period although due to the dose-limiting effect of the lithium this was not always possible. Following the period of *intravenous* GLA administration patients were continued on *oral* GLA (initially at a dose of 3 g/d but increasing to a maximum of 6 g/d if tolerated). Patient characteristics are as shown in Table 4.2.

Inclusion criteria are listed below:

- confirmed pancreatic cancer (clinical or histological diagnosis)
- Karnofsky performance score ≥ 70
- life expectancy ≥ 2 months
- serum albumin concentration ≥ 30 g/l

- patients not receiving any other form of therapy
- fully informed consent (ethical approval given by Lothian Health Board ethics committee)

Immunological and cytokine assessments were carried out prior to treatment (day 0), at day 5 of the infusion and on completion of the intravenous infusion of GLA (day 10). Thereafter assessments were carried out on a monthly basis. At each assessment peripheral blood mononuclear cells (PBMC) were isolated by differential centrifugation. Thereafter the following immunological and cytokine assessment were carried out:

- spontaneous PBMC [³H]-thymidine uptake
- PHA-stimulated PBMC [³H]-thymidine uptake
- anti-CD3-stimulated PBMC [³H]-thymidine uptake
- spontaneous PBMC TNF production
- endotoxin-stimulated PBMC TNF production
- analysis of lymphocyte subpopulations and activation markers by flow cytometry

Table 4.2   Characteristics of patients undergoing GLA treatment (mean ± SD)

Mean age (years)	57 ± 8
M:F	11 : 7
Weight (kg)	60 ± 11
% weight loss	16 ± 10
Albumin (g/l)	38 ± 5
Stage of disease	II 5 III 6 IV 7

Administration and monitoring of lithium-GLA

GLA was formulated as the lithium salt and dissolved in 20% ethanol (where each 1 g vial of LiGLA contained 3.85 mmol of lithium in 5 ml total volume). Prior to administration, the GLA was disolved in normal saline to give a total volume of 1 l and infused at a constant rate over 24 h with daily alterations in the dose depending on (a) the experimental protocol and (b) the serum concentration levels of lithium. The therapeutic range of lithium is 0.6 to 1.0 mmol/l and during the study the maximum serum levels of lithium which we aimed to achieve was 0.8 mmol/l. The mean daily dose of GLA and corresponding serum concentrations of lithium are shown in Fig. 4.2. The mean maximum dose of GLA was 7.6 g against a desired maximum dose of 10 g/d. In some instances ($n =9$), the serum lithium levels precluded achieving the maximum desired dose of GLA.

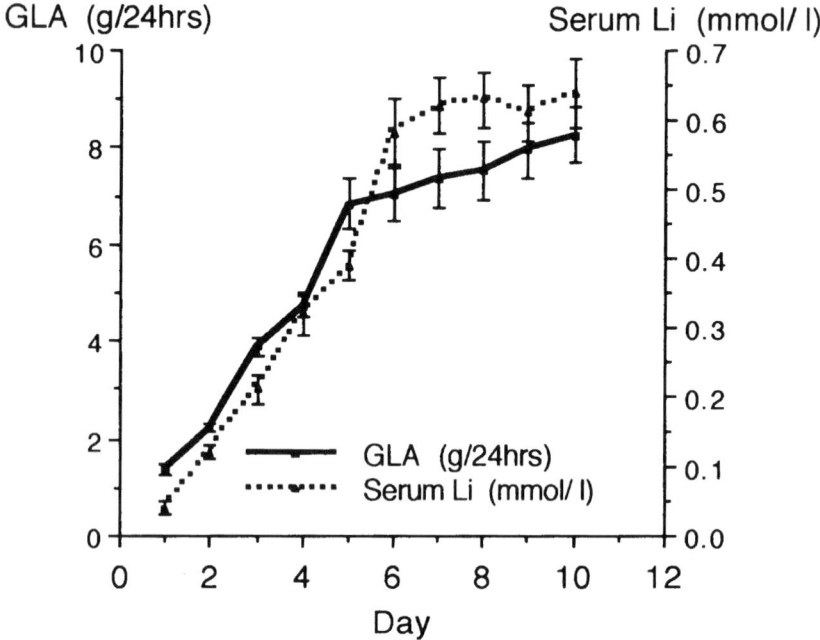

Fig. 4.2   Daily dose (mean ± SEM) of intravenous lithium-GLA (g/24 h) and corresponding serum lithium concentration (mmol/l).

RESULTS

Side-effects and complications

The side-effects and complications that occurred during intravenous GLA therapy are summarised in Table 4.3.

Initially GLA was infused through a peripheral line. However, the first two patients treated developed marked thrombophlebitis. A decision was made to change to central venous infusion of GLA. In subsequent patients (n =16) there were two episodes of subclavian vein thrombosis. Following the first episode 5000 units of heparin/d was added to the GLA infusion but this did not prevent a further thrombosis occuring in the next patient treated. Thereafter 10 000 units of heparin/d was added to the GLA and there were no further episodes of venous thrombosis.

Culture-proven line sepsis occurred in four patients. In two this was only apparent on culturing the central line tip following the completion of intravenous therapy. The other two patients developed clinically obvious infection towards the end of their intravenous therapy and required both removal of the central line and intravenous antibiotics.

Table 4.3   Complications that occurred during intravenous lithium GLA therapy ($n = 18$ patients)

Complication	n
Thrombophlebitis	2
Subclavian vein thrombosis	2
Line sepsis	4
Haemataria	4
PV bleeding	1
Polyuria + polydipsia	1

Haematuria occurred in three patients and was self-limiting in all of them. It occurred following a large incremental increase in the daily dose of GLA. The dosage regimen was subsequently modified to increase GLA more gradually and no further episodes of haematuria have been observed.

One patient had polyuria and polydypsia which is a known side-effect of lithium and one patient had a transient episode of vaginal bleeding.

Thirteen of the 18 patients went on to receive oral GLA. Mild nausea and occasional vomiting occurred in seven of these patients. This resolved on reducing the dose of GLA in two patients and required eventual withdrawal of the capsules in five patients.

Fatty acid profiles

The composition of plasma and red cell membrane phospholipids (analysis kindly performed by Scotia Pharmaceuticals plc) in the pancreatic cancer patients ($n = 10$) prior to starting GLA treatment in relation to those of a large non-cancer group of controls are shown in Fig. 4.3. In general, there were no major differences in plasma phospholipids whereas red cell membrane phospholipid ratios revealed a significantly higher proportion of the saturated and monosaturated fatty acids and a significantly lower proportion of PUFAs in the pancreatic cancer patients.

The changes in the fatty acid profile of the plasma and red cell membrane phospholipids following intravenous infusion of GLA and subsequent administration of oral GLA are shown in Figs 4.4 and 4.5. GLA treatment resulted in a significant decrease in oleic acid (by 17%) and linoleic acid (by 28%) in the plasma phospholipids fraction. The level of EPA also fell significantly (by 41%) following GLA administration. In contrast, the plasma phospholipid levels of dihommo-gamma-linolenic acid (the immediate metabolite of GLA) and arachidonic acid increased significantly during treatment with GLA by 218% and 28% respectively (Fig. 4.4).

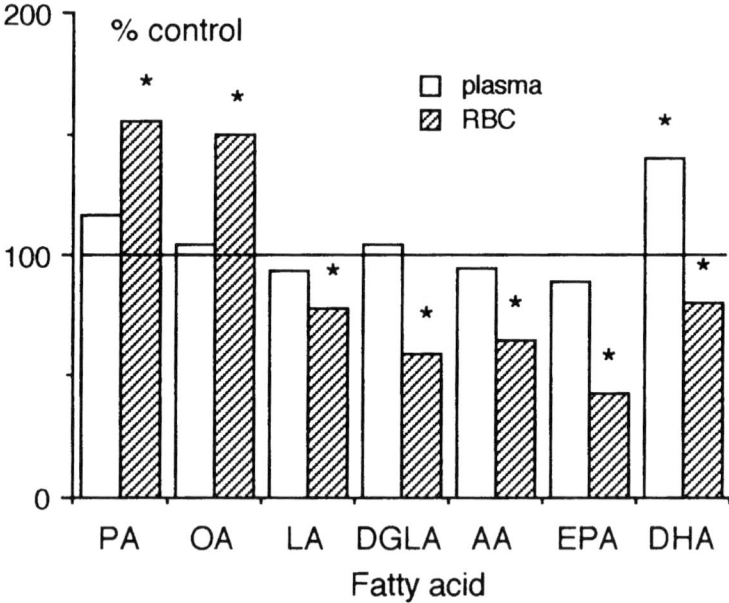

Fig. 4.3   Plasma phospholipids (□) and red cell membrane phospholipids (▨) of pancreatic cancer patients (*n* =10) prior to GLA treatment. Results are expressed as a percentage in comparison with controls (*n* =319). The fatty acids palmitic acid (PA), oleic acid (OA), linoleic acid (LA), dihommogamma-linolenic acid (DGLA), arachidonic acid (AA), eicosapentaenoic acid (EPA) and docosahexaenoic acid (DHA) are shown. *Percentage value versus control; *P*<0.01 (Mann–Whitney U-test).

The changes in red cell membrane phospholipids were less marked. Only dihommo-gamma-linolenic acid changed significantly, increasing by 295% (Fig. 4.5). However, it is likely that when such analysis is carried out after a longer period of GLA treatment that the changes seen in the plasma phospholipid levels at 1 month will be reflected in the membrane phospholipid levels.

T-cell function and cytokine production

The changes in T-cell function observed during GLA treatment are shown in Table 4.4. There was a significant increase in PBMC spontaneous thymidine uptake during the intravenous GLA treatment period and this continued whilst the patients were on oral GLA. PHA-stimulated T-cell thymidine uptake increased slightly at the end of intravenous GLA therapy but was not significantly increased during the period of oral GLA treatment. In contrast, anti-CD3 stimulated T-cell thymidine uptake, although not significantly increased during the phase of intravenous GLA, was significantly increased after 4 weeks of oral GLA. Lymphocyte subsets and markers of activation remained unchanged throughout the infusion period (Fig. 4.6).

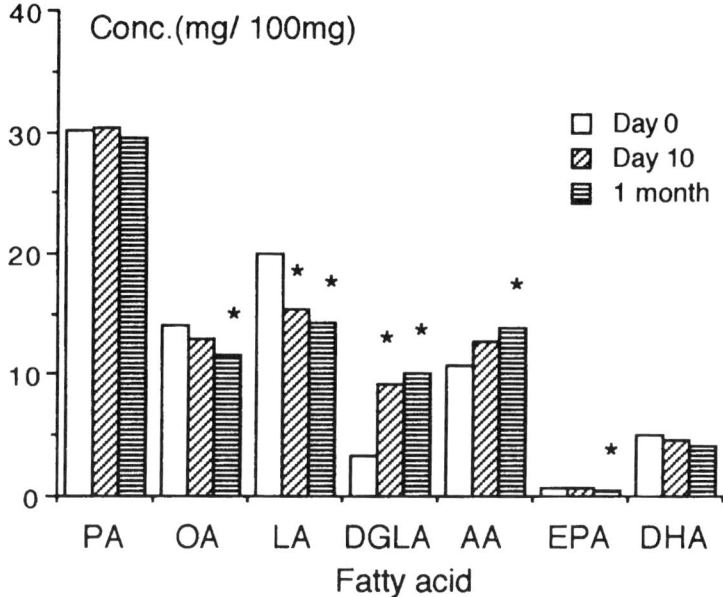

Fig. 4.4   Changes in plasma phospholipids following GLA treatment (n =10). The relative concentration of fatty acids (mg/100 mg) prior to treatment (day 0), at day 10 and at 1 month are shown for palmitic acid (PA), oleic acid (OA), linoleic acid (LA), dihommogamma-linolenic acid (DGLA), arachidonic acid (AA), eicosapentaenoic acid (EPA) and docosahexaenoic acid (DHA). *Relative concentration versus pre-treatment value; $P<0.01$ (Student's paired t-test).

Table 4.4   Spontaneous, PHA-stimulated and anti-CD3 stimulated uptake of [³H]-thymidine by PBMC of pancreatic cancer patients (n =18) during GLA treatment (mean ± SEM of counts/min/10^5 cells)

	Pre-treatment	Day 10	1 month
Spontaneous uptake	606±37	2927±858*	971±114**
PHA-stimulation	86534±8945	109141±8743	106387±12180
Anti-CD3-stimulation	28823±8181	54450±11944	64387±13413**

*Day 10 vs pre-treatment P <0.01; **1 month vs pre-treatment, P < 0.01, Student's paired t-test.

The production of TNF by PBMC both spontaneously, and in response to endotoxin, during GLA treatment is shown in Table 4.5. There was a significant decrease in the amount of TNF produced spontaneously by isolated PBMC following treatment with intravenous and oral GLA. Endotoxin-stimulated TNF production followed a similar pattern but the trend was not statistically significant.

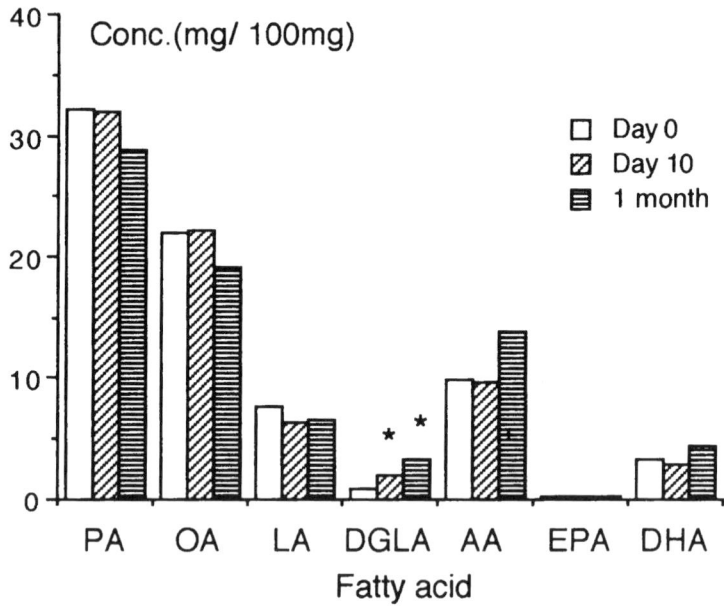

Fig. 4.5 Changes in red cell membrane phospholipids following GLA treatment (*n* =10). The relative concentration of fatty acids prior to treatment (day 0), at day 10 and at 1 month are shown for palmitic acid (PA), oleic acid (OA), linoleic acid (LA), dihommogamma-linolenic acid (DGLA), arachidonic acid (AA), eicosapentaenoic acid (EPA) and docosahexaenoic acid (DHA). *Relative concentration versus pre-treatment value; *P*<0.01 (Student's paired *t*-test).

Table 4.5   Spontaneous and endotoxin-stimulated TNF production by PBMC of pancreatic cancer patients (*n* =18) during GLA treatment (mean ±SEM, pg/ml/10^5 cells)

	Pre-treatment	day 10	1 month
Spontaneous TNF	864±220	1776±512	183±49*
Endotoxin-stimulated TNF	4847±701	8304±1218	3430±706

*1 month vs pre-treatment, *P* <0.02; Student's paired *t*-test.

Duration of survival

Due to the considerable difficulties inherent in imaging accurately the pancreas, survival rather than tumour response rate was used as the clinical end-point in this study. The median survival of the group (*n* =18) was 7.5 months. This is similar to the survival of the treatment group in a previous trial of combined chemotherapy in pancreatic cancer carried out in Edinburgh (Leonard et al 1992). In the latter study the median survival of the treatment group was 8 months as opposed to 3.5 months in the untreated controls. Clearly, because the present GLA study is an

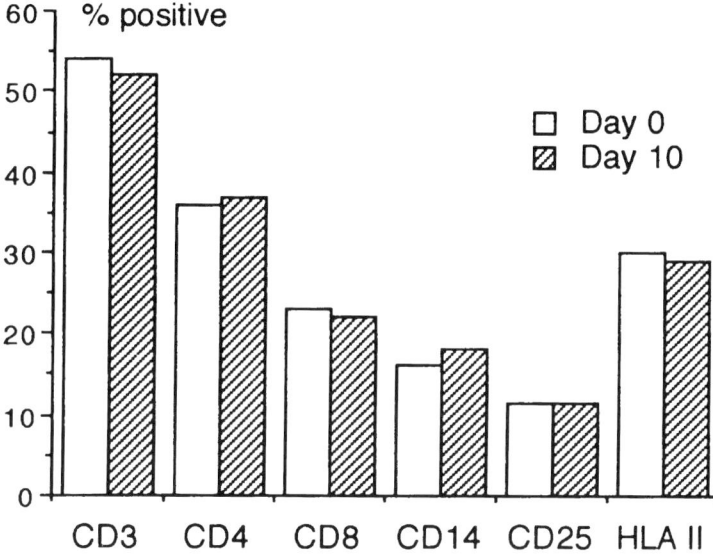

Fig. 4.6   T-cell subpopulations and activation markers following intravenous lithium GLA. The relative percentage of total T-cells (CD3), helper T-cells (CD4), cytotoxic/suppressor T-cells (CD8), monocytes (CD14) and the relative expression of the IL-2 receptor (CD25) and the HLA class II molecule (HLA II) prior to GLA (day 0) and following GLA (day 10) are shown. No changes were statistically significant (Student's paired *t*-test).

uncontrolled open phase II trial, it is impossible to comment on any survival benefit which might be associated with GLA therapy in pancreatic cancer but it would be fair to say that it is relatively free of side-effects and appears to be comparable with conventional combined chemotherapy in terms of patient survival.

ACKNOWLEDGEMENTS

This work has been supported by grants from the Cancer Research Campaign and the Melville Trust for the Care and Cure of Cancer. The GLA was kindly supplied by Dr David Horrobin, Scotia Pharmaceuticals plc and the antibodies were supplied by Drs P. Beverley and K. Guy.

REFERENCES

Beck SA, Smith KL, Tisdale MJ 1991 Anticachectic and antitumour effect of eicosapentaenoic acid and its effect on protein turnover. Cancer Research 51: 6089–6093
Begin ME, Das UN, Ells G, Horrobin DF 1985 Selective killing of human cancer cells by polyunsaturated fatty acids. Prostaglandins, Leukotrienes and Medicine 19: 177–188
Begin ME, Ells G, Das UN, Horrobin FD 1986 Differential killing of human carcinoma cells by n-3 and n-6 polyunsaturated fatty acids. Journal of the National Cancer Institute

USA 77: 1053–1062

Calman KC 1982 Cancer cachexia. British Journal of Hospital Medicine 26: 28–34

Calmus Y, Spielman D, Mendy F et al 1985 Effect of 1.2g of gamma-linolenic acid/day supplementation on membrane arachidonic acid content and on cellular immunity in cirrhotic patients. Gastroenterologie Clinique et Biologique 9: 2

Cancer of the Pancreas Task Force Group 1981 Staging of cancer of the pancreas. Cancer 47: 1631–1637

Carter DC 1989 Cancer of the pancreas. Current Opinions in Gastroenterology 5: 716–722

Cerra FB, Lehman S, Konstantinides N, Konstantinides F, Shronts EP, Holman R 1990 Effect of enteral nutrients on in vitro tests of immune function in ICU patients: a preliminary report. Nutrition 6: 84–87

De Wys WD 1986 Weight loss and nutritional abnormalities in cancer patients: incidence, severity and significance. In: Nutritional support for the cancer patient. Baillière Tindall, London pp 251–261

Dippenaar N, Booyens J, Fabbi D, Katzeff I E 1982 The reversibility of cancer: evidence that malignancy in melanoma cells is gamma-linolenic acid deficiency-dependent. South African Medical Journal 62: 505–509

Endres S, Ghorgani R, Kelley VE et al 1989 The effect of dietary supplementation with n-3 polyunsaturated fatty acids on the synthesis of interleukin-1 and tumour necrosis factor by mononuclear cells. New England Journal of Medicine 320: 265–271

Fearon KCH 1992 The mechanisms and treatment of weight loss in cancer. Proceedings of the Nutrition Society 51: 251–265

Fugiwara F, Todo S, Imashuku S 1983 Anti-tumour effect of gamma-linolenic acid on cultured human neuroblastoma cells. Prostaglandins, Leukotrienes and Medicine 23: 311–320

Gough DB, Winstanley FP, Fearon KCH, Carter DC 1992 Regulation of TNF production in healthy humans and in patients with cancer. Archives of Surgery 127: 713–717

Karmali RA, Marsh J, Fuchs C 1984 Effect of omega-3 fatty acids on growth of a rat mammary tumour. Journal of the National Cancer Institute 73: 457–461

Karmali RA, Reichel P, Cohen LA, Terano T, Hirai A, Tamura Y, Yoshida S 1987 The effects of dietary omega-3 fatty acids on the DU-145 transplantable human prostatic tumour. Anticancer Research 7: 1173–1180

Leonard RCF, Cull A, Stewart ME, Knowles G, Carter D C, Palmer KR 1992 Chemotherapy for pancreatic cancer significantly prolongs survival and quality of life is unimpaired. British Journal of Cancer 65: (Suppl 16) abstract 8

Monson JRT, Ramsden C, Guillou PJ 1986 Decreased interleukin-2 production in patients with gastrointestinal cancer. British Journal of Surgery 73: 483–486

Pritchard GA, Jones DL, Mansel RE 1989 Lipids in breast carcinogenesis. British Journal of Surgery 76: 1069–1073

Wica MS, Liotta LA, Kidwell WR 1979 Effects of free fatty acids on the growth of normal and neoplastic rat mammary epithelial cells. Cancer Research 39: 426–435

Williamson RCN 1988 Pancreatic cancer: the greatest oncological challenge. British Medical Journal 296: 445–446

5. The treatment of carcinoma of the pancreas by lithium gamma-linolenate

P.D. Reynolds Q. Tuffnell A. Lee J. O. Hunter

INTRODUCTION

Carcinoma of the pancreas develops insidiously, progresses relentlessly and is virtually always fatal. In a smaller number of cases surgical resection is possible, but in the majority, no treatment is presently available. The mean survival after diagnosis in patients undergoing palliative surgery, is less than 6 months (Broons & Culebras 1976). Gamma-linolenic acid has been shown to inhibit the growth of several lines of human tumour cells in vitro, and to produce regression of human tumours implanted into mice (Horrobin 1990). Preliminary studies have suggested that it may prolong survival in otherwise untreatable gastro-intestinal malignancies (Manolakas & Van der Merwe 1992). This paper describes the results of trials of both oral and intravenous administration of lithium gamma-linolenic acid (LiGLA) in patients with carcinoma of the pancreas.

PATIENTS AND METHODS

Patients admitted to the trials had been shown to be suffering from carcinoma of the pancreas by CT or MRI scanning, or by histology obtained at laparotomy. They were of either sex, aged 18–80, and were required to have a Karnofsky Performance status of >70%. Patients with carcinoma of the ampulla of Vater were excluded, as were those who had undergone a triple by-pass. Those receiving systemic hormone or chemotherapy for their condition were also excluded, as were any who were taking systemic lithium salts.

Study 1 (oral administration)

This was a double-blind, escalating dose, randomised placebo-controlled study. LiGLA/GLA concentrate (PN 2505, HGC, EF5) was supplied as enteric-coated capsules containing 375 mg gamma-linolenic acid and lithium salt, 87.5 mg linoleic acid, 5 mg lithium ion, with antioxidants, 0.25 ascorbyl palmitate and 0.1 mg citric acid. The placebo were enteric-coated tablets of identical appearance containing 500 mg sunflower oil and the same anti-oxidants.

Capsules were taken twice daily after meals. The dose was initially 4 twice a day, but after 2 weeks this was increased to 6 twice a day and finally after a further 2 weeks to 8 twice a day, which dose was maintained for the remainder of the trial. Returned medication was counted at each assessment visit to assess patient compliance. Such visits occurred monthly for the first 2 months, then 2-monthly for the next 4 months and 3-monthly thereafter.

The primary efficacy parameter was patient survival after the initial diagnosis, but the effect on the patients' quality of life was also assessed.

Study 2 (intravenous administration)

This was an open, uncontrolled study of LiGLA administered either via peripheral vein or through a central line.

LiGLA (PN 5601) was supplied in 5 ml amber glass ampoules dissolved in 20% aqueous ethanol, with 0.05% ascorbyl palmitate and 1% citric acid as anti-oxidants. Unopened ampoules were stored at 4°C in the dark.

LiGLA was dissolved in 0.9% saline as a sterile intravenous infusion, which was mixed very gently to avoid foaming. For the first 2 d patients received a continuous infusion of 2 g in 1 l. The following 2 days the dose was 5 g in 24 h and for the remaining 6 d, if possible, 10 g of LiGLA was given.

During this period serum lithium levels were monitored at least once every 12 h and often 6 hourly at first. The concentration in the plasma of lithium was not allowed to rise above 0.7 mmol/l. Patients were closely monitored for haemolysis and haematuria and treatment was temporarily suspended if this appeared before reintroduction at a lower dose.

After 10 days of intravenous therapy patients were maintained on oral therapy at a dose of 16 capsules daily.

The primary efficacy parameter was patient survival after initial diagnosis, and the patients' quality of life was again assessed.

RESULTS

Study 1

14 patients were admitted to the study. These were randomly allocated to active or placebo treatment and seven were included in each group. There were five females (aged 67–78 years, mean 72.6 years) and nine males (aged 48–78 years, mean 62.5 years).

The stage of disease is shown in Table 5.1. Five patients from each group were in stage 1, two on active treatment were in stage 3 and the remaining two patients in the placebo group were in stages 2 and 4 respectively.

The survival of the patients in the two groups was compared. In the active group survival ranged from 12 to 548 d with a mean of 154.7 d, the median being 63 d. Placebo group survival ranged from 34 to 146 d with a mean of 103.2 days and a median of 100 d. There was no statistically significant difference between the two groups.

The quality of life questionnaire was completed for all the patients in the active group and for four in the placebo group.

Preliminary analysis revealed no significant difference between the two groups although the patients surviving longest not surprisingly scored the most highly.

Table 5.1   Disease stages in Study 1

Stage	Characteristics	Active treatment	Placebo
1	Tumour >2 cm in greatest dimension.	1	3
	Tumour extends to duodenum, bile duct or peripancreatic tissue	4	2
2	Tumour extends directly to stomach, spleen, colon or adjacent large vessels	0	1
3	Regional lymph nodes metastasis	2	0
4	Distant metastasis	0	1

Study 2

19 patients were considered for inclusion in the study. Eight were excluded for the reasons given in Table 5.2. One had previously received oral LiGLA and was therefore excluded from further analysis. The 10 patients remaining included six men and four women aged 52 to 73 years. Two were given LiGLA by peripheral line and received only 10 g and 12 g respectively. Eight were treated via a central line, seven for the full period of 10 days. These received 28–68 g of LiGLA in total (mean 48 g). The maximum daily dose achieved ranged from 6 d to 10 g. One patient was only treated for 6 d because she developed a urine infection. Her total dose was 23 g LiGLA.

Table 5.2   Exclusion criteria for Study 2

19 patients considered
8 excluded
2 declined
2 follow-up impractical
1 treated surgically
1 aged >80 years
2 Karnofsky <70%

Intravenous LiGLA therapy was largely uncomplicated when it was administered by central line. Treatment had to be temporarily stopped in four patients because the plasma lithium concentration rose above 0.77 mmol/l. Eight patients developed haemoglobinuria but this was easily controlled by reducing the dosage and by increasing the dilution of the LiGLA. No problems with coagulation occurred.

Five of the six patients treated for 10 days intravenously subsequently went on to oral therapy but one declined to continue as she felt too unwell to take 16 capsules daily. The patient who suffered the urinary infection also declined oral treatment.

Four of these have since died after 420, 360, 60 and 30 d respectively (mean 217.5 d). Two are still alive at 60 and 90 days. A significant relationship was discovered between the length of survival and the total dose of lithium-GLA ($r = 0.638$, $P = 0.024$).

Quality of life data for these patients is not yet complete.

DISCUSSION

Even though the oral capsules contained GLA in a highly concentrated form, the large number required to provide an adequate daily dose proved too many for most of the patients treated in Study 1. Because of the difficulties encountered by all clinicians in diagnosing carcinoma of the pancreas at an early stage, many of these patients were already extremely ill at presentation. The effort involved in swallowing 16 capsules a day was simply too much for them to cope with, particularly when many had to take other medication to control pain or for coexisting diseases. It is therefore difficult to be sure exactly how effective this treatment may have been and there was no significant difference in the survival between the group of patients treated with LiGLA and that treated with placebo.

Nevertheless, two patients survived for 548 and 219 d respectively, and these were both taking active LiGLA. It is difficult to disprove the suggestion that their longer survival was a consequence of a superior state of health at the time of the initial diagnosis. The numbers involved in this trial were too small to eliminate this possibility. However, these patients both felt greatly improved after starting LiGLA therapy and provided the main justification for attempting to increase GLA levels and improve the clinical condition of these patients by administering LiGLA intravenously.

The intravenous administration of LiGLA presents difficulties as it is likely to produce thrombosis in peripheral veins even when given together with heparin. Fewer difficulties were encountered when it was given through a central line. Furthermore, problems may arise from LiGLA producing haemolysis and haemoglobinuria or the plasma level of lithium rising to toxic levels.

Haemolysis presented few difficulties in this study and by means of careful surveillance of the plasma concentration of lithium, no problems were encountered from lithium toxicity. In the majority of patients we were able to achieve full doses of LiGLA over a 10 day period with a total administered dose ranging from 28 to 68 g.

The survival of the patients treated intravenously has varied between 2 months to a maximum of 14 months. It is difficult to assess the effectiveness of this treatment as many patients were accepted into the study who already had metastatic disease. However, as in study 1, patients with uncomplicated carcinoma of the pancreas felt very much better after LiGLA therapy. In view of the lack of alternative therapy, the prolonged survival for over a year in two patients, and the relative infrequency of side effects encountered, it now seems justifiable to undertake a careful controlled trial of intravenous LiGLA in patients with carcinoma of the pancreas.

REFERENCES

Brooks JR, Culebras JM 1976 Cancer of the pancreas – palliative operation, Whipple procedure or total pancreatectomy? American Journal of Surgery 131: 516
Horrobin DF 1990 Essential fatty acids, lipid peroxidation and cancer. In: Horrobin DF (ed) Omega-6 essential fatty acids. Pathophysiology and roles in clinical medicine. Wiley–Liss, New York, pp 351–378
Manolakas G, Van der Merwe CF 1992 Adjuvant per os administration of gamma-linolenic acid (GLA) in advanced untreatable gastrointestinal malignancies prolongs survival. Hellenic Journal of Gastroenterology 5: (Suppl); 207

6. Survival of patients with pancreatic cancer treated with lithium gamma-linolenate in relation to the dose administered: a combined analysis of the Edinburgh and Cambridge studies

K. C. H. Fearon   J. S. Falconer   J. A. Ross   D. C. Carter
P. D. Reynolds   Q. Tufnell   J. O. Hunter

INTRODUCTION

Pancreatic cancer is usually rapidly fatal. In published controlled trials, the median survival times for the untreated control groups have been 63 d (Mallinson et al 1980), 90 d (Keating et al 1989) and 122 d (Bakkevold et al 1990). In published trials of patients treated with various chemotherapy and radiotherapy regimens, median survivals have ranged from 85 d (Casper et al 1992) to 312 d (Mallinson et al 1980) with an overall median of 160 d. The improvements in survival have been so modest and the side effects so important that few authors have felt able to recommend implementation of the regimen studied.

Lithium gamma-linolenate (EF13, Scotia Pharmaceuticals) is a new anticancer agent based on the effects of gamma-linolenate in selectively killing cancer cells of many different types without harming normal cells (Begin et al 1986). When given intravenously, plasma levels of EF13 are readily monitored by assaying the lithium ion. We have conducted an open study in patients with inoperable pancreatic cancer with an estimated life expectancy of more than 2 months and a Karnofsky performance score of 70% or more.

PATIENTS AND RESULTS

Patients received an intravenous (i.v.) infusion of EF13 diluted in isotonic saline. The rate of infusion was increased over the first 5 d and then maintained at up to 10 g/d for a further 5–7 d. The main complication of the i.v. infusion was rapidly reversible haemolysis caused by the detergent action of gamma-linolenate. However, this could be reduced by slowly increasing the dose so that plasma lithium levels remained below 0.7mmol/l. Peripheral infusions of EF13 caused local venous thrombosis but this could be avoided by infusion into a central vein with an appropriate regimen of heparinization. There were no other important side effects. After completing the infusion, patients were offered oral EF13 up to a maximum of 6 g/d. Approximately 60% of the patients received some oral therapy but in about half the dose had to be reduced or treatment stopped because of nausea and/or diarrhoea.

48 patients have been treated with total i.v. doses ranging from 6 g to 80 g. The lowest i.v. doses were in patients given peripheral venous infusions and who developed venous thrombosis, while the highest doses were given depending on patient tolerance and on our increasing confidence in the methods of infusion and in the absence of serious side effects.

The overall median survival is 158 d and the median survival of those with confirmed histology is 146 d. These survival times are higher than in untreated controls and similar to those reported in previous chemotherapy or radiotherapy trials but without the major side effects. Since this was not a randomized study, we have sought evidence for a dose/survival relationship. Because oral therapy was given less consistently and because the longer patients survived the more oral therapy they were likely to receive, we have restricted this analysis to the cumulative i.v. dose given. Mean and median survival times for patients who received cumulative doses of 0–40 g, 40–60 g and 60–80 g are shown in Table 6.1. Survival of patients who received the highest dose was significantly longer than survival in the lowest dose group ($P =0. 0084$) or in the lowest and intermediate groups combined ($P =0.0081$, Mann–Whitney test).

Table 6.1 Censored mean and estimated median survival times in days in 48 patients with non-resectable pancreatic cancer treated with three different dose ranges of lithium gamma-linolenate (0–40 g, $n =11$, one alive: 40–60 g, $n =15$, four alive: 60–80 g, $n =22$, nine alive)

		Cumulative dose					
	n	Mean (0–40 g)	Median (20 g)	Mean (40–60 g)	Median (50 g)	Mean (60–80 g)	Median (70 g)
All	48	124	89	174	169	270	358
Cambridge	21	87	81	150	168	244	351
Edinburgh	27	168	84	222	179	296	363
Without distant metastases	30	214	162	231	340	326	453
With distant metastases	18	49	59	108	78	143	113

Censored means assume that all patients are dead and are particularly conservative for the high dose group. Estimated medians were calculated using a Cox proportional hazards model and show survivals at the mid-point dose level in each group.

A number of factors may influence survival in a study of pancreatic cancer. These include the presence or absence of distant metastases, sex, the presence or absence of histological confirmation, the centre and the dose of the therapeutic agent being administered. These factors and their first order interactions were entered into a Cox proportional hazards model with regard to their effect on survival. The model showed that only two factors had a significant effect on survival, the presence or absence of distant metastases (P =0.0001) and the dose of lithium-GLA (P =0.0077). None of the interactions was significant. Sex (P =0.52), centre (Cambridge or Edinburgh, P =0.15) and the presence or absence of histological confirmation (P =0.28) had no significant effects. A separate regression analysis including only patients with histologically confirmed cancer showed a highly significant positive relationship between dose of EF13 and survival time from diagnosis (r =0.55, $P<0.005$, n =24). There was no indication of any plateauing of the dose/survival relationship at the highest doses used.

COMMENT

The estimated median survival in patients receiving 70 g of EF13 (358 d) is over three times longer than untreated patients, more than twice as long as the median survival in all the published chemotherapy trials and longer than the previously reported longest median survival in any trial. There was also evidence of improved quality of life. The Karnofsky performance score, after 1 month of EF13 treatment when almost all patients were still alive, was improved or unchanged in 54% of the high dose group, compared to only 27% in the lower dose groups. At 1 month, 50% of the high dose group had unchanged or increased weight, as compared to only 12% in the other groups.

These results must, however, be qualified by the observation that many other factors may influence the duration of survival of patients with pancreatic cancer. These include age, performance status and nutritional/metabolic status. Clearly within a small group of patients such factors may bias results which otherwise appear to depend on the tolerance of a novel chemotherapeutic agent. Lithium gammalinolenate may be an important new anti-cancer agent with unusually low toxicity. Higher doses, repeated courses of treatment and co-administration with other therapies may produce improved survival. A prospective randomized trial is being planned.

REFERENCES

Bakkevold KE, Pettersen A, Arnasjo B, et al 1990 Tamoxifen therapy in unresectable adenocarcinoma of the pancreas and the papilla of Vater. British Journal of Surgery 77: 725–730
Begin ME, Ells G, Das UN, et al 1993 Differential killing of human carcinoma cells

supplemented with n-3 and n-6 polyunsaturated fatty acids. Journal of the National Cancer Institute 77: 1953–1962

Casper ES, Schwartz GK, Johnson B, et al 1992 Phase II trial of edatrexate in patients with advanced pancreatic adenocarcinoma. Investigational New Drugs 10: 313–316

Keating JJ, Johnson PJ, Cochrane AMG, et al 1989. A prospective randomised controlled trial of tamoxifen and cyproterone acetate in pancreatic cancer. British Journal of Cancer 60: 789–792.

Mallinson CN, Rake MO, Cocking JB, et al 1980 Chemotherapy in pancreatic cancer: results of a controlled, prospective, randomised, multicentre trial. British Medical Journal 281: 1589–1591

7. Unsaturated lipids as modulators of radiation damage in normal tissues

J.W. Hopewell   G.J.M.J. van den Aardweg   G.M. Morris
M. Rezvani   M.E.C. Robbins   G.A. Ross   E.M. Whitehouse

INTRODUCTION

In the planning of a patient for radiotherapy, consideration has to be given to the risk of any adverse morbidity that may result from damage to those normal healthy tissues unavoidably included within the treatment volume. These considerations can frequently limit the maximum dose of radiation that might be given to a tumour and thereby affect the likelihood of controlling the malignant lesion. Several approaches are being tried in an attempt to improve the therapeutic ratio in radiotherapy. In addition to modifications in radiotherapy fractionation schedules, attempts have largely focused on the use of agents either to enhance the radiosensitivity of tumour cells, specifically by overcoming the problem of resistant hypoxic cells in solid tumours, or alternatively to selectively protect normal tissues using so called 'radioprotectors'. Such approaches, have as yet, achieved only limited success (Dische 1992, Overgaard et al 1992) and have in themselves often been hampered by the toxicity of some of the agents used (Blumberg et al 1982, Overgaard et al 1989).

An alternative and promising approach is the utilization of interventional treatments after radiation exposure which are directed at modulating steps in the cascade of events leading to the expression of normal tissue damage. This could selectively reduce normal tissue morbidity without compromising tumour cell kill; in therapeutic terms total radiation doses could be increased without an increased risk of morbidity thereby enhancing tumour cell kill and increasing the probability of local disease control. Such approaches using various biological response modulators (BRMs) could bring significant clinical benefits.

The use of growth factors, in overcoming problems associated with a number of acutely responding normal tissues, has been proposed. It has been shown that neutropaenia and the resultant increased risk of infection can be reduced by the administration of granulocyte colony-stimulating factor (G-CSF) following conventional chemotherapy (Bronchud et al 1987). This has provided a rationale for the use of more intensive chemotherapy regimens which may bring considerable benefits to patients

88

with advanced cancer with possible increased cure rates when combined with other modalities. Haematopoietic growth factors also have a role to play in the treatment of radiation accident victims (Gale & Butturini 1990), although supportive care to inhibit the effects of secondary and tertiary factors may in some cases be sufficient to allow recovery in the primary site of damage, i.e. the bone marrow.

Although acute changes in skin, oral mucosa and bowel are important considerations after radiotherapy the major concern is the risk of late tissue morbidity occurring many months, even years, after the completion of therapy. In recent years the effects of various agents, which might be termed BRMs, have been tested in experimental systems. Some of these agents which, unlike growth factors, may act predominantly on the secondary and tertiary cascade of changes, have been demonstrated to significantly ameliorate the expression of late radiation-induced normal tissue damage. These include the use of the angiotensin-converting enzyme (ACE) inhibitor, captopril, effective in reducing radiation damage to the lung (Ward et al 1992) and kidney (Robbins & Hopewell 1986, Cohen et al 1992), the orally active haemorrheological agent, pentoxifylline (PTX), in cutaneous tissues (Dion et al 1989), and the iron chelating agent, desferrioxamine, in the spinal cord (Hornsey et al 1990). For a review see Hopewell et al (1993a).

The precise mode of action of any of the above BRMs, which may interact by several pathophysiological pathways, has still to be elucidated. However, a potential major pathophysiological pathway involved in the development of radiation damage to many normal tissues would appear to be related to alterations in eicosanoid metabolism. In vitro and in vivo studies of radiation effects on the vasculature, damage to which is frequently linked to the evolution of radiation late effects (Hopewell et al 1993a), indicate an initial increase in prostacyclin (PGI_2) followed by a long-term reduction lasting many months (Sinzinger et al 1984, Eldor et al 1989, Rubin et al 1991), although thromboxane (TXA_2) production appears to be unaffected (Allen et al 1981). The resulting imbalance in eicosanoids reported in the lung (Ward et al 1992) and kidney (Weshler et al 1987) after irradiation may adversely influence many vascular functions. Moreover, increases in prostaglandins (PGs) and leukotrienes (LTs) may have a role to play in the expression of acute radiation damage in normal tissues, such as the gut and oral mucosa (Abdelaal et al 1989, Cole et al 1993).

Unsaturated essential fatty acids (EFAs) are known to be important as precursors of eicosanoids (Willis 1981) but also have a significant role with respect to the structure of cell membranes, where they regulate fluidity and flexibility. They also effect the function of membrane related proteins such as receptors, ion channels and those proteins associated with secondary messenger systems (Horrobin 1992a).

The above observations suggested that modifications in EFA levels might have a beneficial effect on the expression of radiation damage in tissues by correcting for the imbalances in eicosanoid metabolism that develop in normal tissues as a consequence of exposure to ionising radiation. The n-6 EFA gamma-linolenic acid (GLA) has been shown to increase the production of the monoenoic prostanoids, PGE_1 and TXA_1. PGE_1 has a number of desirable physiological activities; it is anti-inflammatory, anti-aggregatory and a potent vasodilator (Zurier 1990).

TXA_1 produces none of the harmful side effects of TXA_2. Moreover, GLA results in the formation of 15-OH-dihomogammalinolenic acid (15-OH-DGLA), an inhibitor of the production of LT inflammatory mediators (Horrobin & Manku 1990). In addition, the n-3 EFA eicosapentaenoic acid (EPA) tends to increase the production of trienoic PGs at the expense of the dienoic pathway.

To assess the ability of EFAs to ameliorate radiation-induced injury of normal tissues, the effects of two orally administered oils So-1100, containing linoleic acid (LA) and GLA and So-5407, containing EPA in addition to LA and GLA, were evaluated. Results were compared with animals receiving a 'placebo' oil, So-1129, which contained a similar amount of LA to the other two 'active' oils but no GLA or EPA. The main EFA in the diet is LA but the most important constituents of all membranes are the metabolites dihomogammalinolenic acid (DGLA) and arachidonic acid (AA). The conversion of LA to GLA is slow and rate limiting, especially in humans. The differences between the three oils used will allow, to some extent, an evaluation of the role of EFAs in the modulation of radiation-induced normal tissue injury.

The effects of radiation on selected normal tissues in the pig have been examined. Both early and late changes in skin have been assessed, since its response to radiation is similar to that of other epithelial tissues and the assay methods used produce highly reproducible data (Hopewell & van den Aardweg 1988). Pig skin is also very similar to human skin in terms of its structure and response to radiation (Hopewell 1986). The response of the cervical spinal column was assessed since this is a critical normal tissue at risk in the treatment of head and neck tumours, where overdosage can result in paralysis. In addition, the response of the kidney was evaluated. The kidney is one of the most sensitive of the normal tissues at risk of developing radiation-induced morbidity following abdominal treatments. The development of total body irradiation, prior to bone marrow transplantation, has also led to several recent reports of renal dysfunction (Lawton et al 1991, Lonnerholm et al 1991, van Why et al 1991), and thus radiation-induced nephropathy represents a major limiting factor in cancer therapy.

EXPERIMENTAL DESIGN

Female pigs of the Large White strain were used in these studies. In investigations involving the evaluation of both early and late damage to the skin, pigs of approximately 14 weeks of age were used (22–25 kg body weight); for studies involving the kidney and spinal cord, mature 40–45-week old animals were used (110–125 kg body weight). For all experimental procedures pigs were anaesthetized with a mixture of ~70% oxygen, ~30% nitrous oxide and 2% halothane (Dickinson & Hubbard 1990).

Skin studies

Groups of animals were allocated to receive the active oils So-1100 and So-5407 or a placebo oil So-1129 according to the protocols in Table 7.1. Oils were given orally for 4 weeks prior to irradiation and for 10–16 weeks after the completion of irradiation with single or fractionated doses of $^{90}Sr/^{90}Y$ β-rays, unless otherwise stated.

Table 7.1. Experimental design for studies involving the irradiation of pig skin with single or fractionated doses (20 F/28 d) of $^{90}Sr/^{90}Y$ β-rays

Irradiation schedule	Experimental group	Oil	Daily dose (ml)	Number of animals
Single dose	A	So-1100	1.5	4
	B	So-1100	3.0	6
	C	So-1100	6.0	4
	D	So-5407	3.0	2
	E	So-1129	3.0	2
	F	So-1129	6.0	4
	G	So-1100	3.0	2*
	H	So-1100	3.0	2†
	I	So-1129	3.0	2*
	J	So-1129	3.0	2†
20 F/28 d	K	So-5407	3.0	4
	L	So-1129	3.0	4

*Oils only given for 4 weeks prior to irradiation.
† Oils only given for 10 weeks after irradiation.

One week prior to irradiation, skin sites, 16 per flank on each pig, were marked out by tattooing with India ink. The sites to be irradiated were 25 mm in diameter with 40 mm between sites. Irradiation was with β-rays from 22.5 mm diameter $^{90}Sr/^{90}Y$ plaques (Amersham International, UK) at a dose rate of ~3.0 Gy/min measured at 16 μm depth. Irradiations with single doses were in the range 20–40 Gy for animals receiving 'active' oils and 20–34 Gy for animals receiving the 'placebo' oil. Fractionated irradiation involved five fractions/week over 4 weeks (20 fractions) to total doses of 69–109 Gy ('active' oil) or 53–93 Gy ('placebo' oil).

Following irradiation, the severity of the acute skin reactions was assessed at weekly intervals for a period of 10 weeks, by at least three observers. Skin sites were examined to assess the presence or absence of bright red erythema and/or moist desquamation. Dose-effect relationships for these two reactions were established by assessing the percentage of skin sites that showed these responses at each dose over the time course of the acute skin reaction. These data were analysed using probit analysis and ED_{50} (±SE) values, defined as the dose which caused bright red erythema and/or moist desquamation in 50% of the skin fields irradiated, calculated as a means of comparing the different treatment schedules.

Pigs in which skin sites were irradiated with single doses that received oils, 'active' or 'placebo', for a period of 16 weeks after irradiation (i.e. Groups A–F) and those that only received oils prior to irradiation (Group G and I) had their skin reactions assessed for a further period of 6 weeks (weeks 10–16). The severity of the later dermal reactions was compared on the basis of the dose-related incidence of dusky/mauve erythema and of dermal necrosis (van den Aardweg et al 1988).

In addition to the assessment of acute epithelial and later dermal reactions, in one group of pigs receiving So-5407 (Group K) and another receiving So-1129 (Group L) an evaluation of the effect of the oils on cell proliferation in the unirradiated epidermis, from rump sites, was undertaken. The local, in vito, labelling of epidermal cells in DNA synthesis was achieved by the intradermal injection of 0.1 mCi of [³H]-labelled thymidine according to the method of Morris & Hopewell (1985). Biopsies were taken at 40 min after this pulse labelling and fixed in Bouin's fluid. Autoradiographs, stained with Mayer's haematoxylin, were prepared from 5 μm sections cut from paraplast-embedded tissue and were examined using a ×40 objective to determine the labelling index of cells in the basal layer, as described previously (Morris & Hopewell 1985). The number of cell layers, within the viable epidermis was also quantified. Biopsies were taken prior to and at intervals of 2, 4, 8, 12 and 16 weeks after the start of the daily administration of oils.

Spinal cord studies

A total of 10 mature pigs were included in this study, five received So-5407, the remainder So-1129. Oils were given orally, 12 ml/day, after irradiation for a period of 20 weeks. Irradiation was to a 10 cm length of the spinal cord using parallel opposed beams from a ⁶⁰Co-therapy unit at a dose rate of ~35 cGy/min and a source-to-surface distance (SSD) of 72 cm. The upper margin of the irradiation field was at the junction of cervical vertebrae 1 and 2.

Animals were examined at regular intervals after irradiation for signs of paralysis. Once confirmed, they were killed and the irradiated segment of cord removed and fixed in formal acetic for subsequent histological investigation.

Kidney studies

A total of 12 mature pigs were used in this study. Starting 6 weeks prior to irradiation, four pigs received 10 ml/d of either So-5407 or So-1129; this dosage was maintained for 16 weeks after irradiation. The remaining four pigs received no oils. Both kidneys of all 12 pigs were irradiated with a single dose of 9.8 Gy ^{60}Co γ-rays at a dose rate of ~70 cGy/min.

The glomerular filtration rate (GFR) of each kidney was determined prior to, and at 8, 12, and 16 weeks after irradiation using ^{99m}Tc-diethylene-triamine-pentaacetic acid (^{99m}Tc-DTPA) renography (Robbins 1984, Robbins et al 1985). Renal biopsies were also taken at 9 and 16 weeks after irradiation using a 4.5 inch Tru-cut biopsy needle. Two to three cores of tissue were obtained from one kidney, in each pig, at each time interval. The cores were immediately placed in ice-cold Trump's glutaraldehyde fixative and subsequently embedded in glycomethacrylate resin. From these resin-embedded tissue samples, 1 μm thick sections were cut and stained with periodic acid–Schiff's reagent (PAS) or methenamine silver for evaluation by light microscopy.

EXPERIMENTAL FINDINGS

Skin studies

The ED$_{50}$ values (±SE) for the endpoints of bright red erythema and moist desquamation, characteristic of the early acute skin reaction, for pigs receiving various doses of the 'active' oil So-1100 and the placebo oil So-1129 are given in Table 7.2. In the largest series of animals which received 3.0 ml of the oils daily, administration of So-1100 as compared with So-1129 for just 4 weeks prior to irradiation had no significant effect on the dose–effect relationship for either the incidence of bright red erythema or moist desquamation. This lack of effect was reinforced by a comparison with historical data for moist desquamation (Hopewell & van den Aardweg 1988), where the ED$_{50}$ (±SE) was 27.32 ± 0.52 Gy, intermediate between the values of 26.00 ± 1.8 Gy and 27.91 ± 1.15 Gy for So-1100 and So-1129, respectively, obtained in the present studies.

Administration of 3.0 ml of oils, daily, for 4 weeks prior to irradiation and over the time course of the acute skin reaction, produced a significant modulation ($P<0.05$) of the radiation response in terms of the incidence of moist desquamation and bright red erythema in animals receiving So-1100 as compared with So-1129. Dose modification factors (DMFs) of between 1.13 and 1.24 were obtained. There was also a suggestion of an effect produced by the 'placebo' oil, So-1129, since the ED_{50} values for both bright red erythema and moist desquamation, when this oil was given over the time course of the reaction, were higher than when this oil was just given prior to irradiation. For moist desquamation, where a comparison with historical control data from pigs receiving no oils is possible, a significant effect of the 'placebo' oil is suggested with DMFs of 1.1 ± 0.04 and 1.14 ± 0.04 when compared with the $-4/+16$ week and $+10$ week So-1129 groups, respectively.

Table 7.2. Variation in the ED_{50} values ($\pm SE$) observed following single doses of $^{90}Sr/^{90}Y$ β-irradiation for the acute skin reaction of bright red erythema and moist desquamation

| Treatment period (weeks) | Oil dose (ml) | $ED_{50} \pm SE$ | | DMF ($\pm SE$) |
		So-1100	So-1129	
Bright red erythema				
$-4/+16$	1.5	35.9 ± 1.2	–	–
-4	3.0	26.81 ± 1.15	29.68 ± 1.68	NS
$-4/+16$	3.0	39.23 ± 0.98	31.76 ± 1.39	1.24 ± 0.06
$+10$	3.0	41.16 ± 3.79	34.44 ± 2.35	1.20 ± 0.14
$-4/+16$	6.0	35.05 ± 1.12	38.71 ± 1.47	NS
Moist desquamation*				
$-4/+16$	1.5	28.3 ± 0.93	–	–
-4	3.0	26.00 ± 1.87	27.91 ± 1.15	NS
$-4/+16$	3.0	33.81 ± 0.8	30.04 ± 1.18	1.13 ± 0.05
$+10$	3.0	31.74 ± 1.08	31.03 ± 1.42	NS
$-4/+16$	6.0	33.44 ± 0.95	31.22 ± 0.94	NS

Either So-1100 or So-1129 were administered daily for various treatment periods. Dose modification factors (DMFs) are quoted ($\pm SE$) when the difference between ED_{50} values for the two oils was significant.
*Historical control value, no oils, ED_{50} ($\pm SE$) 27.32 ± 0.52 Gy.

Further evidence for a 'placebo' effect was supported by the results obtained when pigs were given daily doses of 6.0 ml of each oil; the greater modulation produced by So-1100 relative to So-1129 was not seen. Administration of a lower dose of 1.5 ml of So-1100 modified the expression of the inflammatory bright red erythema response but not the severity of moist desquamation.

For the later dermal reactions of dusky/mauve type erythema, seen 10–16 weeks after irradiations, and ischaemic dermal necrosis, daily doses of 3.0 ml of So-1100 also produced a significant modification in the radiation response when results were compared with those seen in the 'placebo' group (Table 7.3). However, the oil had to be given over the time course of the radiation response to be effective. No significant effect was seen when So-1100 (3 ml/d) was only given prior to irradiation. There was evidence, indicative of a 'placebo' effect, when So-1129 was given both before and after irradiation at a dose of 6.0 ml/d. The ED_{50} values were significantly higher than when the same oil was given at 3.0 ml/d ($P \ll 0.001$) and at this higher dose level there was no significant additional gain obtained from the use of So-1100; DMFs were not significantly different from 1.0 (Table 7.3). For these later dermal vascular reactions, 1.5 ml/d of So-1100 produced a significant modulation of the expression of radiation damage when compared with the combined data for pigs receiving 3.0 ml/d of So-1129. The DMFs of 1.26 ± 0.09 and 1.16 ± 0.08 were not significantly different from those obtained using 3.0 ml/day of So-1100 both before and after irradiation (Table 7.3).

Studies involving the oil So-5407 were only carried out using 3.0 ml/d, given both before and after irradiation. Moreover, effects seen after irradiation with single doses of $^{90}Sr/^{90}Y$ β-rays were compared with those seen after a fractionated irradiation schedule (20 F/28 d). The results of these investigations are given in Table 7.4. For the early endpoint of bright red erythema there appears to be a modification in the response seen when compared with a 'placebo' group for both single and fractionated irradiation. However, the difference in ED_{50} values suggesting DMFs of 1.14 ± 0.08 and 1.06 ± 0.04 only approached statistical significance ($0.05 < P < 0.1$). A significant ($P < 0.02$) modification in response was seen for the endpoint of moist desquamation; the DMF was 1.08 ± 0.03. The DMFs noted following irradiation with both single and fractionated doses using the oil So-5407 were in the same range as that found after single dose irradiation using the oil So-1100.

The suggestion of a 'placebo' effect with So-1129 was also detected after irradiation with fractionated doses; the ED_{50} (±SE) of 80.36 ± 1.91 Gy obtained for moist desquamation was significantly higher ($P < 0.02$) than that of 74.52 ± 2.18 Gy for historical controls (Hopewell & van den Aardweg 1991), where no oils were given: DMF = 1.08 ± 0.04.

The effects of So-5407 on the later dermal reactions could only be studied after single dose exposures, since fractionation of the radiation dose reduces the severity of these responses, specifically after $^{90}Sr/^{90}Y$ exposure. Significant modification of the later dermal reactions was seen after the administration of So-5407 over the time course of the reaction as compared with So-1129. These changes were consistent with DMFs of

1.32 ± 0.13 and 1.2 ± 0.12, for dusky/mauve erythema and ischaemic dermal necrosis, respectively.

Table 7.3. Variation in the ED_{50} values (±SE) for the later dermal reactions of dusky/mauve erythema (DE) and ischaemic dermal necrosis (N) after the administration of either So-1100 or So-1129 for various time periods following irradiation with single doses of $^{90}Sr/^{90}Y$ β-rays

Treatment period (weeks)	Oil dose (ml)	ED_{50} ±SE So-1100	ED_{50} ±SE So-1129	DMF (±SE)
Dusky/mauve erythema (DE)				
−4/+16	1.5	32.96 ± 1.61	—	1.26 ± 0.09*
−4	3.0	26.5 ± 1.3	27.5 ± 1.1	NS
−4/+16	3.0	37.53 ± 1.89	24.84 ± 1.53	1.35 ± 0.11
−4/+16	6.0	37.97 ± 1.82	38.44 ± 2.08	NS
Dermal necrosis (N)				
−4/+16	1.5	40.95 ± 2.12	—	1.16 ± 0.08*
−4	3.0	34.8 ± 1.4	35.0 ± 1.5	NS
−4/+16	3.0	40.64 ± 1.31	35.7 ± 1.55	1.14 ± 0.06
−4/+16	6.0	49.56 ± 3.01	51.93 ± 3.87	NS

DMFs are quoted (±SE) when the difference between the ED_{50} values for the two oils was significant.
*DMFs determined by a comparison with the combined data for 3.0 ml of So-1129.

The changes in the labelling index (LI) of basal cells in the epidermis with time after the administration of both So-5407 and So-1129 are shown in Fig. 7.1. Within 2 weeks of the start of administration of both oils the LI of the basal layer had risen from its normal resting value of ~7% to a value of ~13% with no significant difference between pigs on the 'active' or 'placebo' oils. After 4 weeks, the time of irradiation with single doses or the time of the start of irradiation with the fractionated schedule, there had been a further increase in the LI for animals on So-5407, the LI had increased to 18.6 ± 1.9%, significantly higher than the LI noted in the 'placebo' group ($P<0.05$). By 8 weeks after the start of the administration of oils the LI had declined to ~9% and remained at approximately this level for the remaining 8 weeks of the study. There was no significant difference in the effect between the 'active' and 'placebo' group at 8 and 16 weeks after the start of the administration of the oils.

The increase in the labelling index was associated with an increase in the number of cell layers (hyperplasia) within the viable epidermis (Fig.

7.2); the maximum effect was seen at 4 weeks after the start of the administration of oils. The greatest increase in the number of cell layers was seen in the region of the rete pegs, which increased by $26.7 \pm 11.1\%$ in the pigs receiving So-5407 and by $18.75 \pm 9.8\%$ in the 'placebo' group. In the regions of the epidermis, between rete pegs, the increase was smaller, ~15%. From 8–16 weeks after the start of the administration of oils, the level of hyperplasia had declined but the number of viable cell layers in all parts of the epidermis was still increased, relative to pretreatment values (Fig. 7.2).

Table 7.4.   Variation in ED_{50} values ($\pm SE$) for the acute skin reactions of bright red erythema (C) and moist desquamation (MD) and the later dermal reactions of dusky/mauve erythema (DE) and necrosis (N) after either single (SD) or fractionated doses (20 F/28 d) of $^{90}Sr/^{90}Y$ β irradiation

Irradiation schedule	Reaction type	ED_{50} $\pm SE$		DMF $\pm SE$
		So-5407	So-1129	
SD	C	36.23 ± 1.97	31.76 ± 1.39	1.14 ± 0.08
	MD	34.6 ± 1.85	30.04 ± 1.18†	1.15 ± 0.08
20 F/28 d	C	108.4 ± 2.3	102.6 ± 3.16	1.06 ± 0.04
	MD	87.11 ± 1.83	$80.36 \pm 1.91^{\star}$	1.08 ± 0.03
SD	DE	32.88 ± 2.54	24.84 ± 1.53	1.32 ± 0.13
	N	42.74 ± 3.9	35.7 ± 1.55	1.20 ± 0.12

DMFs are quoted for the comparison between So-5407 and So-1129.
*Historical control value, no oils 74.52 ± 2.18 Gy.
† Historical control value, no oils 27.32 ± 0.52 Gy.

Spinal cord studies

Of the five animals receiving 12 ml of So-1129 a day, from the time of irradiation, four developed paralysis after a latent interval of some 8–12 weeks, an incidence ($80 \pm 17.9\%$) consistent with results obtained for animals that received 22 Gy and no oils (Fig. 7.3). In the five pigs receiving So-5407, only a single animal developed paralysis after a latent interval of 8 weeks. This difference in the incidence of myelopathy between animals receiving So-5407 and So-1129 was highly significant ($P < 0.001$).

Kidney studies

Following kidney irradiation (9.8 Gy) all pigs showed a similar pattern of response; the GFR had declined by 8 weeks after irradiation, with minimal values being found 12 weeks after irradiation. However, the extent of

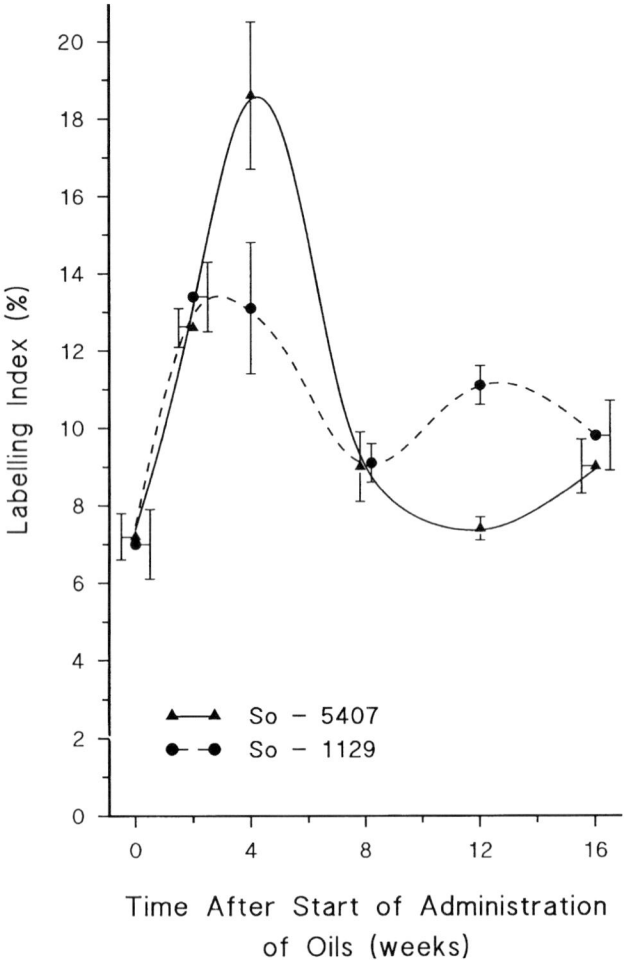

Fig. 7.1.   Time-related changes in the labelling index (%) of cells in the basal layer of the epidermis of the pig after the administration of the oils So-5407 (▲) or So-1129 (●). Error bars indicate ±SE.

the reduction in GFR differed between the various groups of animals. To compare these data, the mean GFR of individual kidneys expressed as a percentage of age-matched controls (Robbins et al 1989), measured between 8 and 16 weeks after irradiation, was established for each treatment group. This analysis showed that the mean GFR for individual kidneys in pigs which received no oils was 27.59 ± 2.19% of age-matched controls. This value was not significantly different from that obtained for pigs receiving So-5407, i.e. 22.26 ± 1.45% of aged-matched controls. However, the mean GFR for individual kidneys in pigs receiving So-1129 was 40.28 ± 3.13% of aged-matched controls, a value significantly higher

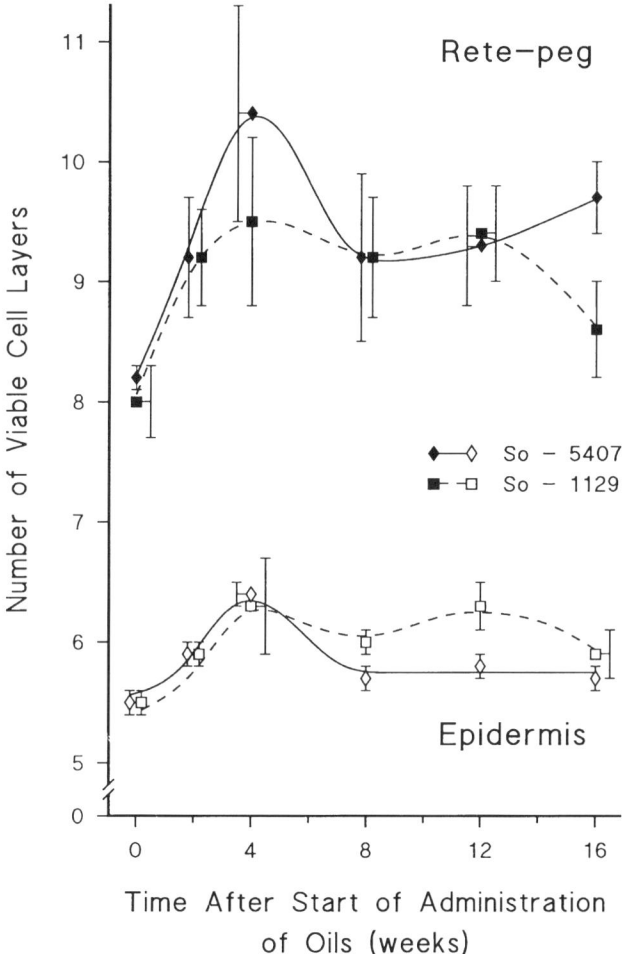

Fig. 7.2.   Time-related changes in the number of cell layers in the viable epidermis of the pig after the administration of the oils So-5407 (◆, ◇) or So-1129 (■, □). Values are given for the epidermis in the region of the rete pegs (◆, ■) and for areas between rete pegs (◇, □). Error bars indicate ±SE.

($P < 0.02$) than that obtained for the other two groups.

These results for functional damage to the kidneys were supported by the histological evaluation of the renal biopsies. In animals receiving irradiation alone glomerular changes similar to those reported previously were observed (Jaenke et al 1993). These included the development of a subendothelial transudation, the accumulation of pericapillary leukocytes, capillary wall thickening and mesangial proliferation. Similar changes were observed in pigs receiving So-5407. However, the extent of these lesions was reduced in pigs receiving So-1129.

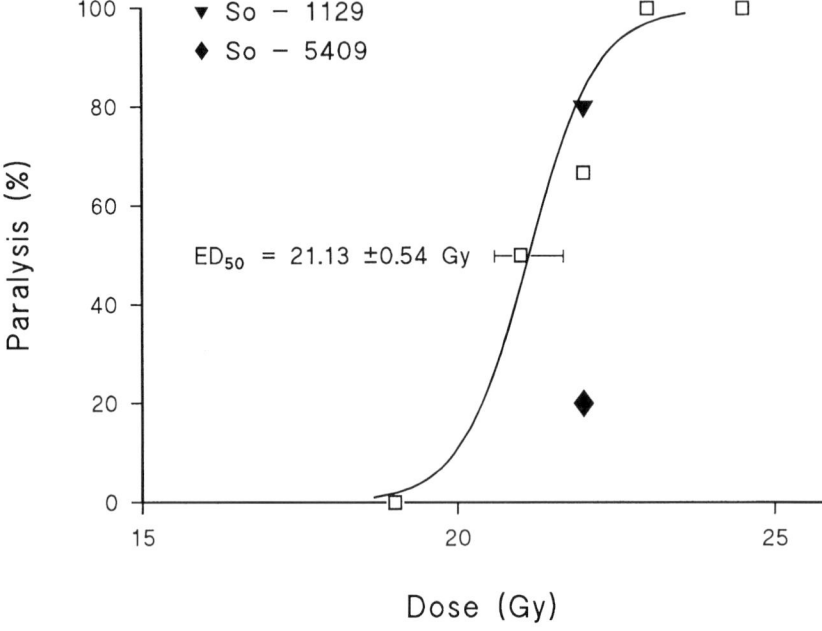

Fig. 7.3.   Dose-related changes in the incidence of paralysis in pigs resulting from radiation-induced myelopathy. The results obtained when pigs were given a 'placebo' oil, So-1129 (▼), and an active oil So-5407 (♦), are compared with the dose response relationship for pigs irradiated over a similar time period that received no oils (□) (Rezvani et al., unpublished). Error bar indicates ED_{50} ±SE.

DISCUSSION

The experimental findings in pig skin clearly illustrate that acute radiation responses can be significantly modified by the administration of EFA metabolites. However, the magnitude of the effect is very dependent on the treatment schedule. In the initial studies with 3 ml of So-1100 daily, as compared with the 'placebo' oil So-1129, oils were given for 4 weeks only prior to irradiation. There were no differences in the acute skin responses, indeed for moist desquamation the ED_{50} values were comparable to those of historical controls (Hopewell & van den Aardweg 1988), suggesting no effect of either oil on the subsequent expression of the radiation damage. This would suggest that the rise in the labelling index of cells in the basal layer after 4 weeks, i.e. ~87% after the administration of So-1129, and the associated increase in the number of viable cell layers had no net effect on the severity of the skin reaction. The potential increase in the number of stem cells at risk at the time of irradiation may have been higher after the administration of So-1100, since an allied 'active' oil, So-5407, which contained small amounts of EPA (1.7%) in addition to GLA (6.9%) and LA (64.5%) resulted in a 2.5-fold increase in the LI after 4 weeks, with a 16–26% increase in the number of viable cell layers. Such an increase in cell proliferation rates produced by So-5407 which contains GLA, a precursor of PGE_1, is consistent with the observation of Levi et al (1990). They reported increased cell proliferation rates and accelerated gastrointestinal repair using exogenous PGE_1. The stimulation of proliferation by the topical application of silver nitrate, induced hyperplasia, and a postulated increase in the number of stem cells prior to irradiaton was used to explain the reduction in oral mucosal reactions seen after radiotherapy (Maciejewski et al 1991).

When the 'active' oils So-1100 and So-5407 were given daily (3 ml) both before and after irradiation both had a beneficial effect when compared with the 'placebo' oil So-1129. This applied to both single and fractionated (20 F/28 d) dose irradiation. The average magnitude of the effect, taking into account the endpoints of bright red erythema and moist desquamation, was represented by a DMF of ~1.13, at the ED_{50} level of effect. Moreover, it also appeared that the administration of the so-called 'placebo' oil, So-1129, had some beneficial effect since when the results obtained in animals after using 3 ml daily doses of this oil were compared with historical control data for moist desquamation for both single and fractionated dose irradiation, significant DMFs of between 1.08 and 1.1 were obtained. Therefore, the true effect of So-1100 and So-5407 would appear to be greater than initially suggested by the present comparative findings. DMF values of 1.27 ± 0.07 and 1.17 ± 0.04 were obtained for single and fractionated doses, respectively, when the results for So-5407 were compared with the historical control data (no oils) for the endpoint of moist desquamation. This represents a clinically very important modulation of the radiation reaction. For comparable single irradiation doses moist desquamation also healed more quickly after the administration of So-1100 (Hopewell et al 1993b).

These benefits gained when the oils were given after irradiation, over the time course of the expression of damage, occurred despite the fact that the initial rise in LI after the administration of either oil, So-5407 or So-1129, declines at least in unirradiated skin between the 4th and 8th week of administration. Thus it is unlikely that the cell kinetic changes explain the observed effects, at least in a simplistic way that can be related to target cell concepts.

The suggestion of a possible effect of the placebo oil, from the use of So-1129 over the time course of the expression of the acute radiation damage, was supported by the results obtained using 6 ml daily of that oil and single dose irradiation. ED_{50} values for bright red erythema and moist desquamation were then increased to comparable levels to those seen using the 'active' oil, So-1100. This 'placebo' effect may reflect the relative importance of LA for the skin (Prottey 1977, Nugteren et al 1985). However, as yet there is little information concerning EFA metabolism in the pig.

The administration of the two 'active' oils, So-1100 and So-5407, 3 ml daily over the time course of the later dermal radiation reaction (10–16 weeks) to single dose irradiation again demonstrated a marked modulation of the reaction when compared with those seen using So-1129. The DMFs for the endpoints of dusky/mauve erythema and dermal necrosis were of the order of ~1.34 and ~1.17, respectively. There was no evidence for any effect of the placebo oil using the 3 ml daily dose, since the ED_{50} values were not significantly different from those obtained for animals that received both oils for only 4 weeks prior to irradiation. It can be assumed that prior treatment with oils produced no modification in the expression of radiation damage to the dermis. However, increasing the dose of both oils to 6 ml, daily, over the time course of the radiation reaction did produce significant evidence for a modulation of the later reactions by the placebo oil, So-1129. Even small doses of So-1100, 1.5 ml daily, over this same period appeared to modulate these later dermal reactions; the effects again appeared to be greater for the inflammatory aspect of the lesion. This suggests a greater ability of GLA to modify the inflammatory aspect of later lesions, possibly through changing membrane structure or by increasing production of PGE_1 and/or reducing LT production (Horrobin & Manku 1990). EFAs are involved in the regulation of platelet and neutrophil adhesion to endothelial cells (Haas et al 1988), reactions which are associated with the expression of late radiation damage in a number of normal tissues (Hopewell et al 1993a). However, the precise mode of action has still to be determined.

The results obtained using So-5407 in reducing the incidence of ischaemic dermal necrosis in the skin of pigs after irradiation with single doses of β-rays could also be shown to be applicable to another late responding tissue, i.e. the spinal cord of the pig. Preliminary results indicated that when So-5407 was administered after irradiation (12 ml daily), over the time course usually associated with the development of radiation myelopathy (van den Aardweg et al 1994) then the incidence of paralysis was significantly reduced. Paralysis results from the selective necrosis of white matter tracks in many animal models of spinal cord injury after irradiation (Powers et al 1992). This selective necrosis of white matter in the irradiated CNS is a function of vascular injury (Hopewell et al 1989). Using 12 ml of the placebo oil, So-1129, produced no evidence of any effect when compared with results for animals that received no oils. This could reflect the dose of this agent used in these larger animals or reduced delta-6-desaturase activity in mature pigs as compared with younger animals. The level of desaturase activity found in samples of the liver of a 26-week-old pig was comparable to those reported in human liver and very different from those in rodents. Pigs of this age are therefore comparable to the human in their ability to desaturate linolenic acid (de Antueno et al, personal communication).

An alternative hypothesis may be derived from the fact that of the 20%

non-aqueous matter made up of EFAs in CNS tissue very little is LA. In the CNS the EFAs are almost entirely those derived from precursors by metabolism in other parts of the body (Horrobin 1992b). Raised exogenous levels of LA have no primary effect on the CNS.

With only limited results available as yet for the spinal cord, it is difficult to estimate the effective modification in the response in terms of an accurate quantifiable DMF. However, assuming a parallel dose effect curve for animals receiving the oil So-5407, a DMF of ~1.1 might be anticipated. Using an alternative approach in a rat spinal cord model, the iron chelator desferrioxamine, with animals maintained on a low iron diet, a similar DMF was obtained (Hornsey et al 1990). Both methods appear to correct for detrimental radiation-induced changes in vascular function.

Given the effective modulation of the expression of late radiation damage to dermal tissue and the spinal cord by So-5407, the failure of the agent to modify the severity of damage to the glomerulus of the kidney, assessed by functional and histological methods, was somewhat surprising. There are many similarities in the pathophysiological mechanisms involved in the development of glomerular lesions in the kidney (Jaenke et al 1993) and in other tissues (Hopewell et al 1993a). Somewhat even more of a surprise was the marked reduction in the impairment of the GFR produced by the use of So-1129. Although an effect of the placebo oil has been demonstrated in the skin this was never in the absence of any effect for the corresponding active oil. Renal tissue has high EFA levels, and PGs of the E series are believed to be of major importance in maintaining the high blood flow to the kidney (Barcelli & Pollak 1985). In addition fish oil which contains EPA, as does So-5407, has been shown to reduce renal damage due to cyclosporin (Elzinger et al 1987). The effective agent in this instance, which reduces radiation-induced injury, contains no EPA. However, the difference in response could well be explained by the way the kidney, in particular the irradiated organ, utilizes EFAs compared with other tissues.

In the studies in kidney the daily dose of both oils was 10 ml. Slightly higher doses were used for mature pigs in which the spinal cord was irradiated. These doses were selected on a somewhat arbitrary basis, since mature pigs are approximately twice the size of female patients being entered into clinical studies. These patients were to receive 6 ml of one of these oils daily (Alcock et al, personal communication) for studies designed to evaluate the modulation of skin damage. A dose of 3 ml daily had been shown to be effective in pig skin (30–38 kg body weight) over the time of expression of damage. However, given the fact that different doses of oils change the response in pig skin and that there are variations in the requirements for EFAs in different tissue, it is obvious that more basic research is required into mechanisms in order to identify optimal treatment schedules for the various tissues at risk of developing adverse morbidity following radiotherapy.

However, these studies do indicate that EFAs can modulate normal tissue responses following radiation and that the DMFs that can be achieved represent a potentially significant clinical effect; a dose of 10% or more being required to produce the same level of normal tissue injury. Such a dose increase would for many tumours, provide a significant improvement in local tumour control by radiotherapy. Furthermore, at the EFA doses envisaged, existing clinical data involving the use of EFAs in other disease conditions have revealed no significant adverse side effects even after administration for periods up to 1 year (Dodge 1990).

Thus the administration of EFAs offers a potentially safe way of reducing radiation-induced normal tissue injury. This taken alongside the tumour cytotoxicity reported in these proceedings, would suggest that EFAs, acting as BRMs, may lead to a significant increase in the therapeutic gain in patients treated for cancer by radiotherapy.

ACKNOWLEDGEMENTS

The authors would like to thank Mr F. Dickinson and Mr N. Hubbard for their expertise in anaesthesia and for the day-to-day care of the animals. Thanks are also due to other members of the Research Institute for help in assessing reactions in the skin studies, Mr J.H. Wilkinson for the preparation of figures and Mrs M. Staff for the careful typing of the manuscript.

REFERENCES

Abdelaal AS, Barker DS, Fergusson MM 1989 Treatment for radiation-induced mucositis. Lancet i: 97
Allen JB, Sagerman RH, Stuart MJ 1981 Irradiation decreases vascular prostacyclin formation with no concomitant effect on platelet thromboxane production. Lancet ii: 1193–1196
Barcelli U, Pollak VE 1985 Is there a role for polyunsaturated fatty acids in the prevention of renal disease and renal failure? Nephron 41: 209–212
Blumberg AL, Nelson DF, Gramkowski M, Glover DJ, Glick JH, Yuhas J, Kligerman MM 1982 Clinical trials of WR2721 with radiation therapy. International Journal of Radiation Oncology, Biology, Physics 8: 561–563
Bronchud MH, Scarffe JH, Thatcher N, Crowther D, Souza LM, Alton NK, Testa NG, Dexter TM 1987 Phase 1/11 Study of recombinant human granulocyte colony-stimulating intensive chemotherapy for small cell lung cancer. British Journal of Cancer 56: 809–813
Cohen EP, Fish BL, Moulder JE 1992 Treatment of radiation nephropathy with captopril. Radiation Research 132: 346–350
Cole AT, Slater K, Sokal M, Filipowicz B, Kurlak L, Hawkey CJ 1993 Elevated rectal leukotriene B_4, thromboxane B_2 and prostaglandin E_2 levels in patients having pelvic radiotherapy. In: Nigam S, Honn KV, Marnett LJ, Walden Jr TL (eds) Eicosanoids and other bioactive lipids in cancer, inflammation and radiation injury. Kluwer Academic Publishers, Boston pp 771–773
Dickinson F, Hubbard N 1990 The Large White female pig in research related to cancer treatment: general husbandry and anaesthesia. Animal Technology 41: 35–41
Dion MW, Hussey DH, Osborne JW 1989 The effect of pentoxifylline on early and late radiation injury following fractionated irradiation in C3H mice. International Journal of Radiation Oncology, Biology, Physics 17: 101–107
Dische S 1992 Radiotherapy, carcinoma of cervix and the radiosensitizer RoO3-8799

(pimonidazole). In: Dewey WC, Edington M, Fry RJM, Hall EJ, Whitmore GF (eds) Radiation research, a twentieth century perspective. Academic Press, London pp 584–589

Dodge JA 1990 Essential fatty acids in cystic fibrosis. In: Horrobin DF (ed) Omega-6 essential fatty acids: pathophysiology and roles in clinical medicine. Wiley-Liss, New York pp 427–435

Eldor A Vladovsky L, Fuks Z, Matzner Y, Rubin DB 1989 Arachidonic metabolism and radiation toxicity in cultures of vascular endothelial cells. Prostaglandins Leukotrienes and Essential Fatty Acids 36: 251–258

Elzinger L, Kelley VE, Houghton DC, Bennett WM 1987 Modification of experimental nephrotoxicity with fish oil as the vehicle for cyclosporin. Transplantation 43: 271–274

Gale RP, Butturini A 1990 The role of hematopoietic growth factors in nuclear and radiation accidents. Experimental Hematology 18: 958–964

Haas TA, Bastida E, Nakamura K et al 1988 Binding of 13-HODE and 5-, 12- and 15-HETE to endothelial cells and subsequent platelet, neutrophil and tumor cell adhesion. Biochimie et Biophysica Acta 961: 153–159

Hopewell JW 1986 Mechanisms of the action of radiation on skin and underlying tissues. British Journal of Radiology (suppl 19): 39–47

Hopewell JW, van den Aardweg GJMJ 1988 Radiobiological studies with pig skin. International Journal of Radiation Oncology, Biology, Physics 14: 1047–1050

Hopewell JW, Calvo W, Reinhold HS 1989 Radiation damage to late-reacting normal tissues. In: Steel GG, Adams G, Horwich A (eds) Biological basis of radiotherapy (2nd edition) Elsevier Scientific, Amsterdam, pp 101–113

Hopewell JW, van den Aardweg GJMJ 1991 Studies of dose-fractionation on early and late responses in pig skin: a re-appraisal of the importance of the overall treatment time and its effects on radiosensitisation and incomplete repair. International Journal of Radiation Oncology, Biology, Physics 21: 1441–1450

Hopewell JW, Robbins MEC, van den Aardweg GJMJ et al 1993b The modulation of radiation-induced damage to pig skin by essential fatty acid. British Journal of Cancer 68: 1–7

Hopewell JW, Calvo W, Jaenke R, Reinhold HS, Robbins MEC, Whitehouse EM 1993a Microvasculature and radiation damage. Recent Results in Cancer Research 130: 1–16

Hornsey S, Myers R, Jenkinson T 1990 The reduction of radiation damage to the spinal cord by post-irradiation administration of vasoactive drugs. International Journal of Radiation Oncology, Biology, Physics 18: 1437–1442

Horrobin DF 1992a Nutritional and medical importance of gamma-linolenic acid. Progress in Lipid Research 31: 163–194

Horrobin DF 1992b The relationship between schizophrenia and essential fatty acid and eicosanoid metabolism. Prostaglandins, Leukotrienes and Essential Fatty Acids 46: 71–77

Horrobin DF, Manku M, 1990 Clinical biochemistry of essential fatty acids. In: Horrobin DF (ed) Omega-6 essential fatty acids: pathophysiology and roles in clinical medicine Wiley-Liss, New York, pp. 21–53

Jaenke RS, Robbins MEC, Bywaters T, Whitehouse E, Rezvani M, Hopewell JW 1993 Capillary endothelium: target-site of renal radiation injury. Laboratory Investigation

Lawton CA, Cohen PA, Barber-Derus SW, Murray KJ, Ash RC, Casper JT, Moulder JE 1991 Late renal dysfunction in adult survivors of bone marrow transplantation. Cancer 67: 2795–2800

Levi S, Goodlad RA, Lee CY, Stamp G, Walport MJ, Wright NA, Hodgson HJF 1990 Inhibitory effect of non-steroidal anti-inflammatory drugs on mucosal cell proliferation associated with gastric ulcer healing. Lancet ii: 840–843

Lonnerholm G, Carlson K, Bratteby LE et al 1991 Renal function after autologous bone marrow transplantation. Bone Marrow Transplant 8: 129–143

Maciejewski B, Zajusz A, Pilecki B et al 1991 Acute mucositis in the stimulated oral mucosa of patients during radiotherapy for head and neck cancer. Radiotherapy and Oncology 22: 7–11

Morris GM, Hopewell JW 1985 Pig epidermis: a cell kinetic study. Cell Tissue Kinetics 18: 407–415

Nugteren DH, Christ-Hazelhof E, van der Beck A et al 1985 Metabolism of linoleic acid and other essential fatty acids in the epidermis of the rat. Biochimie et Biophysica Acta 834: 429–436

Overgaard J, Sand Hansen H, Andersen AP et al 1989. Misonidazole combined with spilt-course radiotherapy in the treatment of invasive carcinoma of larynx and pharynx: report from the DAHANCA 2 study. International Journal of Radiation Oncology, Biology, Physics 16: 1065–1068

Overgaard J, Sand Hansen H, Overgaard M, Jorgensen K, Bastholt L, Berthelsen A, Pedersen M 1992 The Danish Head and Neck Cancer Study Group (DAHANCA) randomized trials with hypoxic radiosensitizers in carcinoma of the larynx and pharynx. In: Dewey WC, Edington M, Fry RJM, Hall, EJ, Whitmore GF (eds) Radiation research, a twentieth century perspective, Academic Press, London, pp 573–577

Powers BE, Beck ER, Gillette EL, Gould DH, LeCouter RA 1992 Pathology of radiation injury to the canine spinal cord. International Journal of Radiation Oncology, Biology, Physics 23: 539–549

Prottey C 1977 Investigation of functions of essential fatty acids in the skin. British Journal of Dermatology 97: 29–38

Robbins MEC 1984 Single injection techniques in determining age-related changes in porcine renal function. International Journal Applied Radiation Isotopes 35: 85–91

Robbins MEC, Campling D, Rezvani M, Golding SJ, Hopewell JW 1989 Radiation nephropathy in mature pigs following the irradiation of both kidneys. International Journal of Radiation Biology 56: 83–98

Robbins MEC, Hopewell JW 1986 Physiological factors effecting renal radiation tolerance: a guide to the treatment of late effects. British Journal of Cancer (suppl VII): 265–267

Robbins MEC, Hopewell JW, Gunn Y 1985 Effects of single doses of X rays on renal function in unilaterally irradiated pigs. Radiotherapy and Oncology 4: 143–151

Rubin DB, Drab EA, Ward WF 1991 Physiological and biochemical markers of the endothelial cell response to irradiation. International Journal of Radiation Biology 60: 29–32

Sinzinger H, Cromwell M, Firbas W 1984 Long-lasting depression of rabbit aortic prostacyclin formation by single-dose irradiation. Radiation Research 97: 533–536

van den Aardweg GJMJ, Hopewell JH, Simmonds RH 1988 Repair and recovery in the epithelium and vascular connective tissue of pig skin after irradiation. Radiotherapy and Oncology 11: 73–82

van den Aardweg GJMJ, Hopewell JW, Whitehouse EM, Calvo W 1994 A new model of radiation-induced myelopathy: a comparison of the response in mature and immature pigs. International Journal of Radiation Oncology, Biology, Physiology (in press)

Van Why SK, Friedman AL, Wei LJ, Hong R 1991 Renal insufficiency after bone marrow transplantation in children. Bone Marrow Transplant 7: 383–388

Ward WF, Molteni A, Ts'ao CH, Kim YT, Hinz JM 1992 Radiation pneumotoxicity in rats: modification by inhibitors of angiotensin converting enzyme. International Journal of Radiatiation Oncology, Biology, Physics 22: 623–625

Weshler Z, Raz A, Rosenmann E, Biran, S, Fuks Z, Eldor A 1987. Thromboxane and prostacyclin production by irradiated and perfused rat kidney. In: Walden TL, Hughes HN (eds), Prostaglandins and lipid metabolism in radiation injury. Plenum, New York, pp 219–224

Willis AL 1981 Nutritional and pharmacological factors in eicosanoid biology. Nutrition Review 39: 289–300

Zurier RB 1990 Prostaglandin E$_1$: is it useful? Journal of Rheumatology 17: 1439–1441

Photodynamic therapy

8. *Meta*-tetra(hydroxyphenyl)-chlorin (*m*-THPC): a second generation photosensitizer for photodynamic therapy: a review

J. C. M. Stewart

INTRODUCTION

Photodynamic therapy (PDT)[1-3] is emerging as an important new procedure for treating malignancy.

The treatment, in short, comprises exogenous administration of a light-absorbing compound which is also called a sensitizer or photosensitizer and which can accumulate in a target tissue. After a delay of hours or days, determined by the kinetics of the sensitizer's distribution, light of wavelength matching its absorption characteristics is directed at the target tissue to photoactivate the sensitizer. This generates free radicals at a rate that overwhelms tissue defences and causes cell death. Neither the sensitizer alone nor light alone has the capacity to generate free radicals at a destructive rate and so are individually inactive as therapies. The combination of both photosensitizer and light is required in the photodynamic process.

Although the concept of PDT has been around for the best part of this century[4] and although light activation of chemicals is an established form of treatment in non-malignant disorders, as in PUVA for psoriasis, it has proved more difficult to develop PDT for cancer largely because no wholly suitable photosensitizers have been available for this purpose.

Photodynamic therapy in cancer is an attractive option for a number of reasons. Thus, it can be used as a single treatment modality or in conjunction with surgery, radiotherapy or chemotherapy depending on circumstances. It can, in principle be made highly selective for cancer by purposefully directing the light at the cancer during the photoactivation process and by using sensitizers which localize in the cancer. This development would represent a considerable therapeutic advance where the tumour is invading vital structures like nerve or vessels and where any treatment by other means is limited if not impossible.

It appears that every tumour cell line of whatever origin, barring only pigmented lesions which may absorb irradiated light excessively, is sensitive to the PDT process. Moreover, the problem of multi-drug resistance which is a serious limitation in conventional oncology does not cross transfer to

PDT[5]; even cell lines exhibiting multi-drug resistance can be killed by PDT. The treatment is wholly without the common side effects of chemotherapy and radiotherapy, such as neutropenia, sickness, hair loss and tissue atrophy. Indeed it can be remarkably atraumatic. Patients who have been conscious while receiving PDT to small tumours have generally noticed little pain or sensation at the time of treatment. Often mild analgesia post procedurally is all that is required; though the amount of pain increases with the size of the tumour treated and strong analgesia may be required after treatment of large lesions. A few days after treatment, the tumour appears necrotic and 2 or 3 weeks later it sloughs off leaving a very clean wound, which re-epithelializes well and does not form scar tissue.

The only consistent side effect of photodynamic therapy is the risk of photosensitization at unwanted sites, especially the skin, following exposure to bright light. The degree and duration of the risk varies with sensitizer and is related to drug kinetics and distribution. This problem can be addressed by keeping the patient out of bright light during the at-risk period and by using sensitizers which do not accumulate in the skin, or are rapidly excreted from the body.

This paper will discuss the basic mechanisms of photodynamic therapy, the properties required of a good photosensitizer, and laboratory and early clinical data obtained with *meta*-tetra(hydroxyphenyl)chlorin (*m*-THPC) – the most promising photosensitizer now in development.

Sensitizers for PDT: mechanism of action and required properties

In PDT, the toxic agent is singlet oxygen, a high-energy reactive oxygen species where electrons have an anti-symmetrical spin, in contradistinction to ground state oxygen, where the electrons have a symmetrical spin. The sensitizer catalyses the production of singlet oxygen from oxygen, potentially with great amplification, depending on the sensitizer's efficiency and providing also tissues are well oxygenated. Availability of oxygen may be a rate-limiting factor in PDT which should not be performed in severely hypoxic conditions. Singlet oxygen can peroxidize unsaturated fatty acids, cholesterol and the indole moiety of histidine and tryptophan, and guanine. Thus all cell structures can be peroxidized and destroyed if they lie close to the site of singlet oxygen generation. In practice though sensitizers tend *not* to localize in the nucleus of the cell so DNA is not directly subjected to the PDT process. This situation is very different from that with normal cytotoxic drugs which are specifically designed to interfere with cell replication. The 'at risk' distance for peroxidation is considered to be around 1 μm or about 1/20th of the diameter of a eucaryotic cell, the distance which singlet oxygen can travel during its lifetime (1–4 μs in aqueous solution)[6,7]

Oxygen needs energy of 94 kJ/mole to raise it from the triplet ground state to the excited singlet state (The unit for measuring energy is the joule. 1 joule is the energy needed to push against a force of 1 newton for 1 metre (1 J= 1 Nm). 1 kilojoule (1 kJ) is dissipated as heat raises 50 cm³ of water by about 5°C.) In photodynamic therapy this energy is obtained from the sensitizer, which itself has been raised to a high-energy state. The process is illustrated in Fig. 8.1. Only sensitizers which can emit more energy than 94 kJ/mol are capable of activating singlet oxygen. This corresponds to a wavelength of approximately 850 nm. It follows that only those compounds which absorb below this wavelength are suitable for photodynamic therapy. (This is a simplification of the actual process of photoactivation. 94 kJ correspond to 1270 nm, so any dye which absorbs at 1270 nm or lower wavelength should theoretically be able to activate oxygen. In practice the light-absorbing compound loses some energy during its conversion to a metastable triplet state before energy is transferred to oxygen. The degree of energy loss varies from compound to compound but it is found that only those which absorb light at 850 nm or lower are efficient sensitizers. Other photophysical properties too are important. Compounds with a short triplet lifetime do not have an opportunity to transfer their energy to oxygen efficiently. The most efficient sensitizer is one which yields one molecule of singlet oxygen for each photon (quantum yield 1) absorbed.)

Another constraint placed upon a sensitizer's suitability is the depth to which the activating light can penetrate tissue. Longer wavelength (red) light can penetrate much more deeply than shorter wavelength (blue/green) light. Red light of around 650 nm for example can penetrate 1 cm of tissue, while light of 400 nm can only penetrate tissue superficially. In practice, sensitizers which absorb in the region of 600–850 nm are likely to be the best as they possess the right energetics for generating

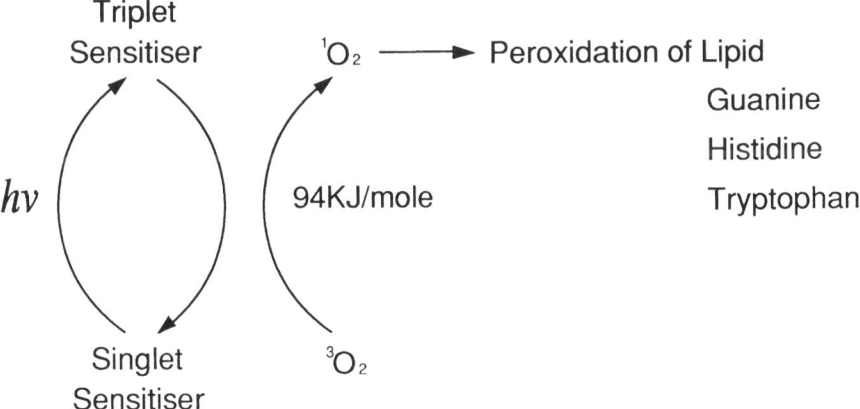

Fig. 8.1. Mechanism of cell destruction.

singlet oxygen and also absorb light at wavelengths which can penetrate tissues to sufficient depth to allow treatment of thick tumours.

Other requirements for a photosensitizer[8] include lack of inherent toxicity, specificity for cancer cells, rapid body clearance to minimize unwanted photosensitization long after the patient has received treatment and good photophysical properties.

Many existing photosensitizers have poor photophysical properties which lead to long treatment times (30 min or longer) in the clinic, a clear disadvantage in clinical practice. Moreover, prolonged irradiation may lead to vessel shutdown and tissue hypoxia[9]. Under these circumstances singlet oxygen is not generated and tumour cells may survive the treatment, only to regrow.

Sensitizers

Compounds of the porphyrin, phthalocyanine and related classes absorb in the 600–850 nm range and so it is principally these that have been assessed for PDT. Figure 8.2, shows the principal peaks of absorption for these classes of compounds and the transmittance of light through tissue at these wavelengths. Porphyrins have a characteristic absorption spectrum of four peaks which include peaks at around 400 nm and 514 nm (as well as 630 nm). Porphyrins thus are particularly interesting as possible sensitizers since irradiation at 514 nm might be preferred over 630 nm for treating the superficial cancers in hollow thin-walled organs like the oesophagus. Light of 514 nm[10] can only penetrate superficially so the PDT process is confined to a thin region and risk of perforation of these organs is lessened. Yet other bands at around 400 nm can be used to induce porphyrin fluorescence which can be used as a diagnostic aid to detect the site of cancer during PDT process.

Haematoporphyrin derivative: a first-generation sensitizer

Haematoporphyrin derivative (HpD)[11,12] is the forerunner of the modern-era photosensitisers. It is made from haematoporphyrin and is a complex mixture of monomeric and polymeric porphyrins, largely uncharacterized[13,14]. Despite the complexity it and a partially purified version, Photofrin, have been widely used to treat cancer with measurable success. Several thousand patients have now received this treatment and high complete response rates have been achieved for early and superficial cancer[15–17] with HpD-mediated PDT. Photofrin is the first photosensitizer to be licensed for any therapeutic use, receiving marketing approval in Canada in April 1993 for the treatment of recurrent superficial papillary bladder cancer. In April 1994 it was licensed in the Netherlands for palliation of certain oesophageal and lung cancers.

HpD is a substance that almost happened by chance[11] and though widely used in photodynamic therapy, it has many limitations in spite of

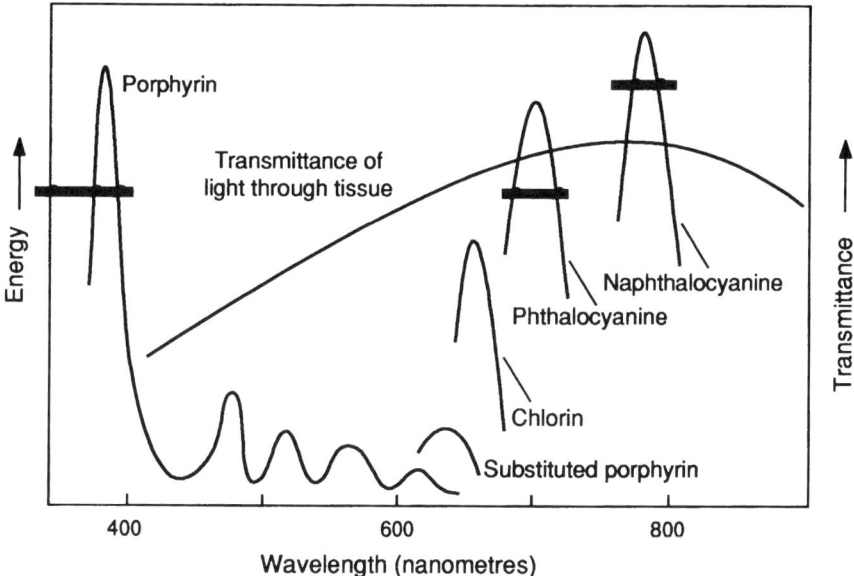

Fig. 8.2. Absorption characteristics of porphyrin, phthalocyanine and related compounds. The amount of light passing through human tissue 1 cm thick, related to absorption by porphyrins.

its successes. The principal disadvantages of haematoporphyrin are its complexity and the lack of detailed knowledge of its active component (or components), its variable but long half-life of ~19 days[6,18] and consequently its prolonged risk to patients of skin sensitization to sunlight. It absorbs at 630 nm, a wavelength at which light does not penetrate tissue deeply, and with a quantum yield of around 0.5 is not a particularly active sensitizer. It is unlikely that HpD will be a suitable sensitizer for tumours which are deeper than 5 mm. Treatment times too can be long, for example doses up to 200 J/cm[2] have been recorded. This can be inconveniently long, and has the added disadvantage that prolonged irradiation may lead to vessel shutdown and tissue hypoxia.

As HpD is, nonetheless, the only sensitizer licensed for therapeutic use, new sensitizers will have to be compared against it for effect.

Second-generation sensitizer: *meta*-tetra(hydroxyphenyl)chlorin (*m*-THPC)

The limitations of HpD have generated an intense search for better photosensitizers loosely referred to as 'second generation sensitizers'. The properties of an ideal sensitizer have been outlined in some detail by Moan[8]. These are that the compound should be a single pure substance since this allows detailed study of pharmacokinetics and distribution within organs and intra-cellularly, have low intrinsic toxicity, selective uptake to cancer cells and good photophysical properties in vivo, whereby there is a high production of singlet oxygen for each photon absorbed by the drug. Many compounds have been proposed and tested. Amongst these one group of compounds, the 5,10,15,20 tetrahydroxyphenyl porphyrins and chlorins[19,20] possess many of the desired characteristics and indeed become close to being ideal sensitizers.

m-THPC (Fig. 8.3) has been selected from this group of compounds for clinical use because of its very high potency as a sensitizer and particular affinity for tumour tissue. Table 8.1 shows the depth of necrosis obtained in a xenograft model, in which groups of plasma cell tumour-bearing mice were sensitized with Photofrin or m-THPC prior to light delivery and the depth of necrosis assessed by histology[19]. Under the experimental conditions of the study in which standard light conditions were used, 0.53 mg/kg of m-THPC produced in excess of 5 mm necrosis. The dose of HpD required for the same depth of necrosis was 96 mg/ml, a factor of approximately 180.

m-THPC has several properties which may explain this potency relative to HpD. Firstly, in keeping with chlorins in general it has a characteristic absorption band at 652 nm. This is well shifted to the red compared with 628 nm, the absorption maximum of haematoporphyrin. The red shift allows irradiated light to penetrate tissue more deeply. Moreover, the

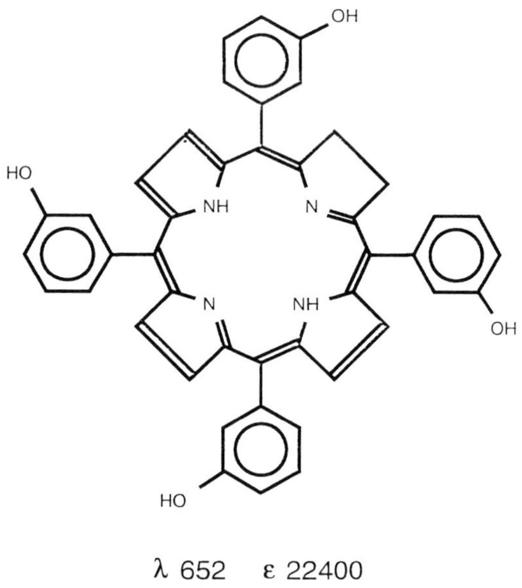

$$\lambda\ 652 \quad \varepsilon\ 22400$$

Fig. 8.3.   Structure of *meta*-tetra(hydroxyphenyl)chlorin.

molar absorptivity (molar extinction coefficient) of *m*-THPC at 652 nm is 22 400 mol^{-1} cm^{-1} [24]. This is much higher than the extinction coefficient for individual components of haematoporphyrin – around 2–3000 mol^{-1} cm^{-1} at 625 nm[13]. The concentration of *m*-THPC in tumour tissue is around 1.5 µg after 24 h[21]. This compares with 4–5 µg/g of tissue for HpD[6]. Finally the quantum yield for *m*-THPC at 0.87 is higher than that for HpD[22] (around 0.5), so it is a more efficient generator of singlet oxygen, mole for mole.

Taken together, these properties could account for much of the difference in activity between the two sensitizers. Other factors such as the site of location within a tumour cell may also be important in determining activity. As yet very little is known about tissue localization of *m*-THPC, but it is known in general that a substance's solubility characteristics can profoundly affect cellular distribution and activity. The more lipophylic compounds localize to cell membranes and seem to be more active[7]. *m*-THPC is very soluble in organic (lipid) solution; it also has amphyllic properties.

Table 8.1.   Depth of tumour necrosis obtained with *m*-THPC and Photofrin II

Dose of sensitizer	Depth of tumour necrosis (mm)	
(mg/kg)	*m*-THPC	PhII
0.136	0.1	—
0.25	2.8	—
0.53	>5.3	—
1.06	>7.3	—
2.125	—	—
4.25	—	—
8.5	—	—
17.0	—	0.0
34.0	—	2.1
48.0	—	3.6
68.0	—	4.0
96.0	—	4.3

Inbred BALB/C female mice were used. Subcutaneous implants of PC6 plasma cell tumour were illuminated above the tumour with a light dose of 10 J/cm^2 and 2–300m W/cm^2 intensity at 650 nm for *m*-THPC or 625 nm for Photofrin II. An Oxford Laser Cu10 copper vapour laser pumping on DL10K dye laser was used. The dye was Rhodamine 640. 24 h after illumination the depth of tumour necrosis was measured on tumour sections on a dissecting microscope, after pre-staining the tumour in the living mouse with Evans Blue. Data from Berenbaum, Ref 19, and Personal Communication.

Selectivity for cancer tissue

Although *m*-THPC is markedly more potent than HpD, mole for mole, such differences are not necessarily an overriding advantage in a sensitizer, since they can be overcome by adjusting dose. The selectivity of the photosensitizer for the tumour, relative to surrounding normal tissue is, however, of prime concern to the operator, since normal tissue may be irradiated during treatment.

Clearly the lower the concentration of sentizer in normal tissue at the time of irradiation the lower the risk of photodamage, and the more selective the treatment. From this would flow the possibility of treating tumours which approximate closely to or invade vital structures. It is hoped that PDT will provide more selectivity than any other measure including radiotherapy, chemotherapy and surgery.

The specificity of m-THPC for tumour tissues has been measured and compared to Photofrin by Berenbaum et al[19,20] using a method of 'damage index'. In this method the tumour and normal tissues of mice were each irradiated under standard lighting conditions and increasing drug doses. Phototoxicity was judged by the appearance of oedema (measured by increase in tissue weight) or necrosis of the test tissue and a damage index is calculated by the following formula:

$$\text{damage index} = \frac{\text{Weight of treated sample} - \text{Weight control}}{\text{Weight control}}$$

It can be seen that a damage index of 1 represents a doubling of weight while a damage index of 0 means no change in weight. Figure 8.4 is a plot of the damage indices for tumour (depth of necrosis) and other tissues (increase in weight or necrosis) obtained over a range of increasing dose of sensitizer. This shows that under the lighting conditions of the experiment 5 mm of tumour necrosis was achieved by m-THPC mediated PDT at a dose level of 0.53 mg/kg for little or no damage to normal tissue. At higher drug dose levels more normal tissue damage occurred. This contrasts with Photofrin II where some normal tissue damage is present at all drug doses, whatever the depth of tumour necrosis.

This result shows that under appropriate operational conditions it is possible to destroy tumour selectively using m-THPC-PDT while there is no 'selective window' for Photofrin II. Some of the selectivity may be explained by differences of drug concentration in tissue at the time of irradiation. The differences appear to be greater for m-THPC than HpD, but the reason for the greater uptake of m-THPC exhibited by cancer cells is not understood.

The above studies were conducted with plasma cell tumours. m-THPC-PDT has also been shown to be active against mesothelioma, squamous cell tumours, colorectal and glioma under experimental conditions, apparently to the same degree of activity as against plasma cell tumours.

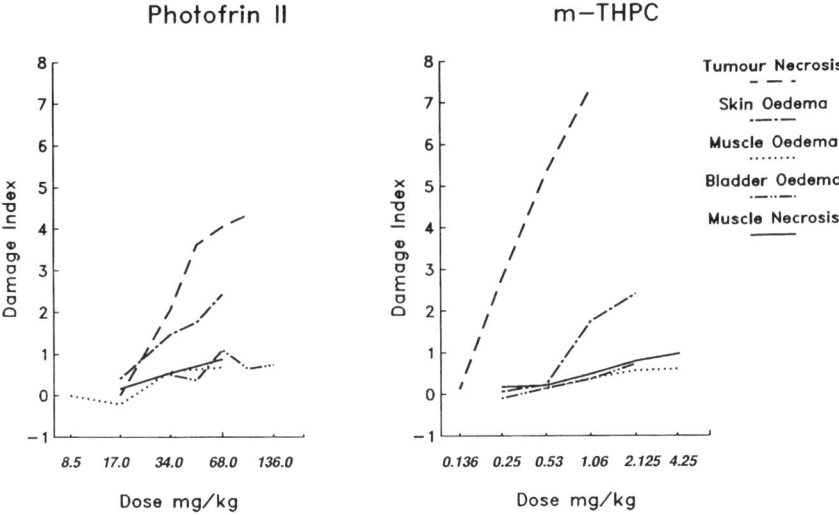

Fig. 8.4. Inbred BALB/C mice of either sex were used to determine tumour necrosis and damage index. The mice were sensitized 1–3 d before illumination. 10 J/cm² of light was applied to each site. Tumour necrosis was determined as detailed in Fig. 2.1. The degree of skin oedema was measured by the increase in weight to a 1cm diameter test site of skin 4 h after exposure. Bladder oedema was measured by increase in weight 1 h after exposure of light to the bladder. Muscle oedema was measured by exposing the hind leg muscle to light and weighing 4 h after exposure. Necrosis was determined by loss of sarcolemmal nuclei 24 h after exposure. (Data from Berenbaum et al, refs 19,20).

CLINICAL STUDIES: CONDITIONS FOR CLINICAL USE

These animal studies established several important principles of *m*-THPC-PDT, namely that it is effective in a wide range of tumours and apparently equally so, under a given set of conditions. This finding is in keeping with the behaviour of photosensitizers in general. Compared to Photofrin II, *m*-THPC is a more potent tumour sensitizer. It is also more selective for tumours than for normal tissue. It is also effective under relatively mild conditions. It takes approximately 2 min to deliver 10 J/cm² of light at an intensity of 100 mW/cm² under which conditions 5–10 mm depth of tumour necrosis is obtained. The short treatment times makes *m*-THPC-PDT more clinically acceptable and has led to early Phase I clinical trials. In these, *m*-THPC-PDT was used adjunctively, during surgery for mesothelioma[21] and alone for the treatment of locally metastased breast cancer[24]. The results from these studies show that 5–10 mm of tumour necrosis is obtained under the same lighting conditions established experimentally. The conditions for clinical use of *m*-THPC-PDT treatment and for HpD-PDT taken from the literature are summarized in Table 8.2. Further studies in gut and head and neck cancer are now in progress.

Many aspects of treatment however, are still not fully settled. In particular the optimum time between drug administration and light administration (the light–drug interval) is not known. It seems for example that with increased intervals there is less normal tissue damage under standard drug dose and light conditions. Drug–light intervals of 48 h, 72 h and 7 d were each used in the Phase I treatments with mesothelioma and breast cancer, but it is not known which of these light intervals or others will be best for most circumstances. Also, light *intensity* rather than *dose* may be profoundly important. Recent animal studies[25] show that the depth of tumour necrosis and therapeutic ratio (damage to tumour v normal tissue) were greatly enhanced by increasing the light intensity from 100 mW/cm^2 to 200 mW/cm^2. Possibly, this can be explained by the dynamics of singlet oxygen generation. Tissue hypoxia due to vasospasm arises during long treatment times[9]. Under such conditions singlet oxygen production falls off too. Shorter treatment times when the tissue is adequately oxygenated is, on the other hand, likely to ensure maximum production of singlet oxygen, and maximum photosensitizing effect.

Table 8.2.   Summary of treatment conditions (clinical)

Sensitizer	*m*-THPC	HpD/Phll
Drug dose (mg/kg)	0.15 – 0.3	2.0 – 5
Wavelength of irradiation (nm)	652	630
Light dose, intensity (cm^2)	20 J, 1–200 mW	40–200J, 1–200 mW
Time of irradiation (s)	100–200	200–2000

The increased photodynamic effect and therapeutic ratio with high intensity light clearly demonstrates that the dynamics of light delivery play an extremely important part in PDT and that as much therapeutic gain may be had from changing light conditions as from changing drug dose. Animal models can only act as a useful guide in selecting the best treatment schedule however, since the tumour is growing in an abnormal milieu in such models, and has an abnormal size proportionate to the size of the animal. It is likely that the best conditions for treatment will only be established during clinical use from carefully constructed protocols.

Future possibilities

It is a regular happening in cancer therapy that new treatments are only first applied to cases where all existing treatments have failed. This is a harsh, though understandable, approach to the problem of cancer therapy. It is important therefore to be realistic about the potential place of *m*-THPC-PDT. For example, PDT is not likely to increase a patient's life expectancy significantly, if distant metastases were present, though it may provide much needed palliation for relief of symptomatic obstruction. On the other hand, effective management of smaller tumours should lead to a complete response to treatment. Probably the depth of tumour (rather than area) is the most prognostic parameter in this respect. With HpD-PDT only tumours of less than 0.5 cm depth can realistically be treated by superficial illumination; the potential for *m*-THPC is much greater. Given good staging facilities, for example by ultrasound or CT, from which the dimensions of a tumour can be precisely determined, and more information about the consistency of *m*-THPC-PDT depth of necrosis, the ease of this treatment should lead to it being the method of choice in many primary tumours.

PDT may also be particularly suited to treating 'field changes' of whole surfaces, for example of the urinary bladder or mouth, where there is widespread dysplastic change or carcinoma in situ. This presents a severe clinical challenge where other treatment options are limited if not impossible. These are very different clinical problems and it is likely that specific treatment conditions will evolve for each after study.

CONCLUSIONS

m-THPC is a potent second generation photosensitizer for photodynamic therapy. It has many properties required of an ideal sensitizer. In particular it is possible to induce tumour necrosis to a depth of 5–10 mm using *m*-THPC-PDT applied for 1–2 min/cm^2 of tumour. These mild conditions make *m*-THPC 'clinically friendly' and potentially the treatment of choice for primary tumours and widespread dysplastic change of some surfaces.

REFERENCES

1. Bock G, Harnett S (eds) 1989 Photosensitizing compounds: their chemistry, biology and clinical use. Ciba Foundation Symposium 146. John Wiley & Sons, Chichester.
2. Henderson BW, Dougherty TJ (eds) 1992 Photodynamic therapy: basic principles and clinical applications. Library of Congress Cataloging in Publication Data. Marcel Dekker Inc, New York
3. Kessel D 1992 Photodynamic therapy and neoplastic disease. Oncology Research 4(6): 219–225
4. Daniell MD, Hill JS 1991 A history of photodynamic therapy. Australian and New Zealand Journal of Surgery 61: 340–348
5. Kessel D, Erickson C 1992 Porphyrin photosensitisation of multi-drug resistant cell types. Photochemistry and Photobiology 55(3); 397–399
6. Henderson BW, Dougherty TJ 1992 How does photodynamic therapy work? Photochemistry and Photobiology 55: 145–157
7. Moan J, Berg K, Kvam E, Western A, Malik Z, Ruck A, Schneckenburger H 1989 Intracellular localization of photosensitizers. In Bock G, Harnett S (eds) Photosensitizing compounds: their chemistry, biology and clinical use, Ciba Foundation Symposium 146 John Wiley & Sons, Chichester, 95–111,
8. Moan J 1990 Properties for optimal PDT sensitizers. Journal of Photochemistry and Photobiology 5(3–4): 521–524
9. Tromberg BJ, Orenstein A, Kimel S, Barker SJ, Hyatt J, Nelson JS, Berns MW 1990

In vivo tumor oxygen tension measurements for the evaluation of the efficiency of photodynamic therapy. Photochemistry and Photobiology 52(2): 375–385

10.   Van Gemert JC, Berenbaum MC, Gijsbers GHM 1985 Wavelength and light dose dependence in tumour phototherapy with haematoporphyrin derivative. British Journal of Cancer 52: 43–49

11.   Lipson RL, Baldes EJ 1960 The photodynamic properties of a particular hematoporphyrin derivative. Archives of Dermatology 82: 508–516

12.   Gregorie HB Jnr, Horger EO, Ward JL, Green JF, Richards T, Robertson HC Jnr, Stevenson TB 1968. Hematoporphyrin derivative fluorescence in malignant neoplasms. Annals of Surgery 167(6): 820–828

13.   Bonnett R, Ridge RJ, Scourides PA, Berenbaum MC 1981, On the nature of 'Haematoporphyrin Derivative.' J.C.S. Perkin 3135–3139

14.   Byrne CJ, Marshallsay LV, Ward AD 1990 The composition of Photofrin II. Journal of Photochemistry and Photobiology B 6: 13–27

15.   Patrice T, Foultier MT, Yactayo S, Douet MC, Maloisel F, Le Bodic L 1990 Endoscopic photodynamic therapy with haematoporphyrin derivative in gastroenterology. Journal of Photochemistry and Photobiology B 6(1–2): 157–165

16.   Monnier Ph, Savary M, Fontolliet Ch, Wagnieres G, Chatelain A, Cornaz P, Depeursinge Ch, Van Den Bergh H 1990 Photodetection and photodynamic therapy of 'early' squamous cell carcinomas of the pharynx, oesophagus and tracheobrochial tree. Lasers in Medical Science 5: 149–169

17.   Jocham D 1992 PDT in bladder cancer Photodynamics Newsletter (ed S.B. Brown issue 5). Media Medica, Chichester

18.   Brown SB, Vernon DI, Holroyd JA, Marcus S, Trust R, Hawkins W, Shah A, Tonelli A 1992 Pharmacokinetics of photofrin in man. In: Spinelli P, Dal Fante M, Marchesini R (eds) Proceedings of the International Conference on Photodynamic Therapy and Medical Laser Applications. Exerpta Medica, London, pp. 475–479

19.   Berenbaum MC, Akande SL, Bonnett R, Kaur H, Ioannou S, White RD, Winifield UJ 1986 meso Tetra (hydroxyphenyl) porphyrins, a new class of potent tumour photosensitisers with favourable selectivity. British Journal of Cancer 54: 717–725

20.   Bonnett R, White RD, Winfield UJ, Berenbaum MC 1989 Hydroporphyrins of the meso-tetra (hyroxyphenyl) porphyrin series as tumour photosensitizers. Biochemical Journal 261(1): 277–280

21.   Ris H-B, Altermatt HJ, Inderbitzi R, Hess R, Nachbur B, Stewart JCM, Wang Q, Lim CK, Bonnett R, Berenbaum MC, Althaus U, 1991 Photodynamic therapy with chlorins for diffuse malignant mesothelioma: initial clinical results. British Journal of Cancer 64: 1116–1120

22.   Patrice T – Personal communication

23.   Ris H-B, Altermatt HJ, Nachbur B, Stewart JCM, Wang Q, Lim CK, Bonnett R, Althaus U 1992 Clinical evaluation of photodynamic therapy with *m*THPC for chest malignancies. In: Spinelli P, Dal Fante M, Marchesini R (eds) Proceedings of the International Conference on Photodynamic Therapy and Medical Laser Applications. Exerpta Medica, London, pp. 421–425

24.   Ris H-B, Altermatt HJ, Stewart CM, Schaffner T, Wang Q, Lim CK, Bonnett R Althaus U 1993 Photodynamic therapy with *m*-tetrahydroxyphenylchlorin in vivo: optimization of the therapeutic index. International Journal of Cancer 55: 245–249

9. Fluorescence imaging and photodynamic therapy with *m*-THPC and Photofrin in a rat skin-fold observation chamber model

N. van der Veen   E. van Leengoed   W. Star

INTRODUCTION

Photodynamic therapy (PDT) is an experimental cancer treatment modality, which uses a photosensitive dye and visible light (Dougherty & Marcus 1992). To date, haematoporphyrin derivative (HpD) is practically the only dye that has been used in clinical PDT. HpD is a mixture of various porphyrins. The amount of active material in HpD depends on the manufacturing procedure. A 'purified' form of HpD, enriched in the photodynamically active fraction has the trade name Photofrin (manufactured by QLT-Phototherapeutics, Canada and Lederle Laboratories, USA). This material is presently the most commonly used photosensitizer for clinical PDT.

A few hours/days after administration of Photofrin, tumour tissue may contain more drug than the surrounding normal tissue. Whether this occurs depends on the type of normal tissue, which itself may also retain a high concentration of Photofrin (e.g. liver). The tumour selectivity of Photofrin combined with its fluorescence offers a means for tumour localization. Selective tumour fluorescence has been demonstrated, e.g. for small superficial human lung (Lam et al 1990) and bladder tumours (Baumgartner et al 1987, Unsöld et al 1990). When (tumour) tissue containing Photofrin is exposed to light of proper wavelength and dose, tissue necrosis occurs within a few days. The (limited) tumour selectivity in the retention of Photofrin results in a certain tumour selectivity of this treatment, which can be enhanced by selective irradiation. Nevertheless, some normal tissue damage always occurs.

Administration of haematoporphyrin derivatives causes transient skin photosensitivity of patients, which may last more than 1 month. After encouraging results had been obtained in the treatment by PDT of various human malignancies many groups have started a search for better photosensitizers. The most important requirement for new photosensitizers, apart from photodynamic efficiency, is reduced skin photosensitivity.

121

Additional advantages would be improved tumour selectivity and maximum light absorption at a longer wavelength than Photofrin, thus increasing the tissue penetration of the activating light. Photofrin is not a single compound, but a mixture of porphyrins including monomers, dimers and oligomers. The monomers show the strongest fluorescence, whereas the dimers and oligomers are the most photodynamically active. Therefore, if selective tumour fluorescence is observed, this does not necessarily mean that the photodynamically active fraction of Photofrin is also selectively retained, and vice versa. An alternative photosensitizer for PDT should therefore preferably be a single compound.

Several improved photosensitizers have already been tested in animal experiments and further improvements are to be expected. In the present paper we will discuss preliminary experimental results on induced tumour fluorescence and photodynamic therapy obtained with *meta*-tetra(hydroxyphenyl)chlorin (Scotia Pharmaceuticals, UK). This drug appears to be a remarkably effective photosensitizer (Bonnet et al 1989, Ris et al 1991, 1993). It also shows highly selective fluorescence of tumour over normal (subcutaneous) tissue in our model system. If skin photosensitivity induced by *m*-THPC would appear to be less than with Photofrin, *m*-THPC could be a promising alternative.

MATERIALS AND METHODS

Animal model

We used 12-week-old female WAG/Rij rats, weighing about 150 g. Observation chambers were prepared in a skin-fold on the back of the rats, according to a procedure described by Reinhold et al (1981). The diameter of visible tissue in the chamber is 9 mm. A chamber could be opened on one side to transplant a syngeneic RMA mammary carcinoma into the subcutaneous tissue in the chamber. Fluorescence and PDT studies were performed when tumours had reached a diameter of 2.5–3 mm, which took about 7 d following transplantation. The animals were kept in a temperature controlled cabinet at 32°C with a 12/12 h light/dark cycle. The elevated ambient temperature determines the temperature of the chamber and is therefore essential for tumour growth. After drug administration the light level in the cabinet was kept below 30 $\mu W/cm^2$. Throughout the experiments, Hypnorm (fluanisol/fentanyl mixture, Janssen Pharmaceutics, Beerse, Belgium) was used as a general anaesthetic.

Photosensitizers

Our experimental results on photodynamic therapy and induced tumour and normal tissue fluorescence with HpD and Photofrin have been reported previously (Star et al 1986, Van Leengoed et al 1990). In the present paper we will briefly summarize the published results, illustrated with typical photographs. For experimental details we refer to the cited papers. *m*-THPC (trade name EF9) was a gift from Scotia Pharmaceuticals Ltd (Guildford, Surrey, UK). The drug was obtained as powder and 5 mg was dissolved in a mixture of 2 g ethanol (96%) and 3 g polyethylene glycol and was diluted with water (PBS) to a volume of 10 ml (concentration 0.5 mg/ml); 1.0 mg/kg was administered i.v. via the tail vein. For injection of 0.3 mg/kg the solution was further diluted to 0.1 mg/ml with the same solvent.

Fluorescence excitation and detection

Fluorescence of Photofrin was excited with 514.5 nm argon laser light at 0.1 mW/cm^2 which is sufficiently low to avoid photodynamic damage by the excitation light. Fluorescence was recorded through a high pass coloured glass filter (RG665). Fluorescence of *m*-THPC was excited at ≈0.1 mW/cm^2 with a 60 nm band of light around 400 nm obtained from a halogen lamp through an interference filter. Fluorescence was recorded around 650 nm through a broad band (40 nm) interference filter.

Fluorescence images were recorded with a CCD video camera equipped with a two-stage image intensifier and a 25 mm Photar macro lens (Leitz). The video images were digitized on a PC-based frame grabber (PC Vision Plus), averaged over 16 frames to improve the signal-to-noise ratio and stored on disk for further processing. The system digitizes 256×256 picture elements (pixels). Average grey scale values of a selected area of interest, i.e. tumour, blood vessel or subcutaneous tissue, were calculated using a pixel measurement programme based on image processing software called TIM (Difa Measuring Systems BV, Breda, The Netherlands).

Photodynamic therapy

The light source was a Spectra Physics model 171 argon laser, pumping a model 375 dye laser with DCM as the lasing medium. For PDT with HpD the laser was tuned to 632 nm (Star et al 1986). In later studies with Photofrin 625 nm was used (Star et al 1990). For PDT with *m*-THPC the wavelength was 652±1 nm. The wavelength was checked with a monochromator. Anaesthetized animals were accomodated on the stage of a Leitz Orthoplan microscope which was heated to keep the body temperature close to normal. Light was transported from the laser with an optical fibre. With a lens and diaphragm a beam was formed of uniform intensity and diameter slightly larger than the diameter of the tissue in the chamber. This beam was projected onto the back of the chamber through the stage of the microscope. The irradiance was 60 or 100 mW/cm^2 in PDT with HpD/Photofrin and 50 mW/cm^2 in PDT with *m*-THPC (See Figs 9.5, 9.6). The layer of tissue in the observation chamber is so thin (0.3–0.5

mm) that a decrease of the fluence rate as a function of depth may be neglected. Indeed, observations on both sides of the chamber showed no difference in damage.

At fixed times during PDT (irradiation interrupted) and up to 7 days after PDT the damage to the vasculature (blood circulation) of tumour and normal tissue was observed, described and photographed. Each observation was translated into a score on a 0–8 scale, i.e. nine levels. A score of 0 indicates no observable damage whereas a score of 8 indicates no observable circulation. A scoring system with five levels was described by Star et al (1986). This was refined by introducing an additional level between each of the five previously defined ones, increasing the total number to nine.

RESULTS

Fluorescence

The results obtained with Photofrin have been reported previously (Van Leengoed et al 1990). Briefly, after administration of HpD or Photofrin (15 mg/kg), in our model enhanced tumour over normal tissue fluorescence never occurred in more than 40% of cases and the optimum ratio was achieved less than 4 h post injection (p.i.). At 24 h p.i. normal tissue

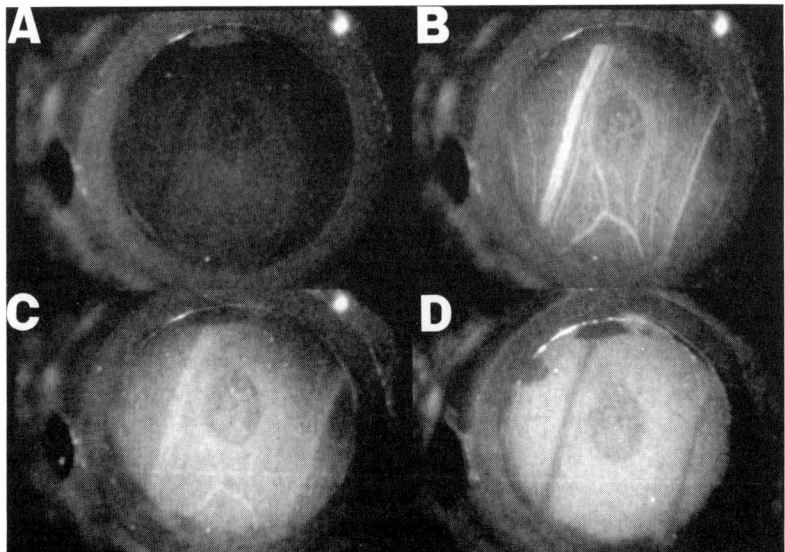

Fig. 9.1. Fluorescence of tumour, normal tissue and blood vessels in the observation chamber model at several intervals after i.v. administration of 10 mg/kg Photofrin. (A) Before drug injection (autofluorescence); (B) at 5 min. p.i. a fluorescence angiogram is clearly visible; (C) 5 h p.i. the fluorescence in the blood vessels has decreased and the tissue fluorescence has increased; (D) 24 h p.i. The two large venules are visible as dark channels. The tumour is visible in the centre.

fluorescence exceeded tumour fluorescence in 60% of cases. Figure 9.1 shows a less favourable example, where no enhanced fluorescence of tumour over normal tissue was observed at any time post injection.

Highly selective tumour fluorescence was always observed following i.v. administration of 1.0 mg/kg *m*-THPC (Fig.9.2). Fluorescence in the blood vessels was not observed except in one case, where a very weak fluorescence angiogram could be discerned shortly and up to 5 h after injection. At that time tumour fluorescence was visible but was also very weak. Figure 9.3 shows the measured tumour and normal tissue fluorescence as a function of time p.i. of 1.0 mg/kg *m*-THPC. Maximum tumour fluorescence occurs 3 days p.i., but the maximum ratio of tumour to normal tissue occurs 1 day p.i. (Fig. 9.4). This ratio subsequently decreases due to increasing normal tissue fluorescence. Remarkably, tissue fluorescence following administration of 0.3 mg/kg *m*-THPC was hardly observable. These measurements were therefore not plotted in Figure 9.3, but only as ratios in Figure 9.4. The decreasing ratio after day zero for 0.3 mg/kg suggests that any increase in tissue fluorescence above the autofluorescence (by not much more than 10%) is larger in the normal tissue than in the tumour.

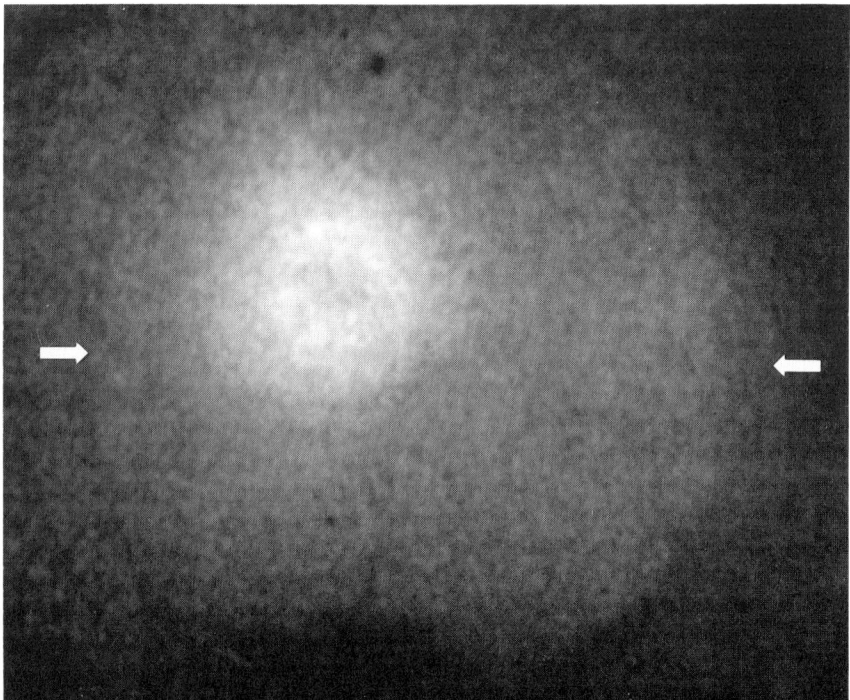

Fig. 9.2. Selective tumour fluorescence in the observation chamber model, 24 h after i.v. administration of 1 mg/kg *m*-THPC, with maximum tumour to normal tissue ratio. Arrows indicate the normal tissue boundary in the chamber. No fluorescence in blood vessels is observed here. The quantitative development of tumour and normal tissue fluorescence as a function of time after drug injection is shown in Figs 9.3. and 9.4.

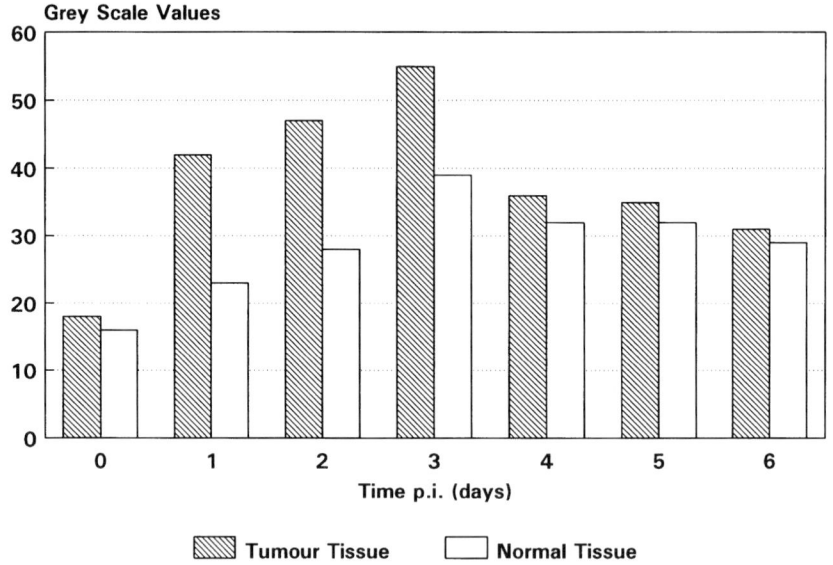

Fig. 9.3. Tumour and normal tissue fluorescence in the observation chamber model as a function of time after i.v. administration of 1.0 mg/kg *m*-THPC (*n*=4). The fluorescence intensity is expressed in arbitrary units using the grey scale levels generated with the image processing software. The values at day 0 are before *m*-THPC injection, i.e. autofluorescence.

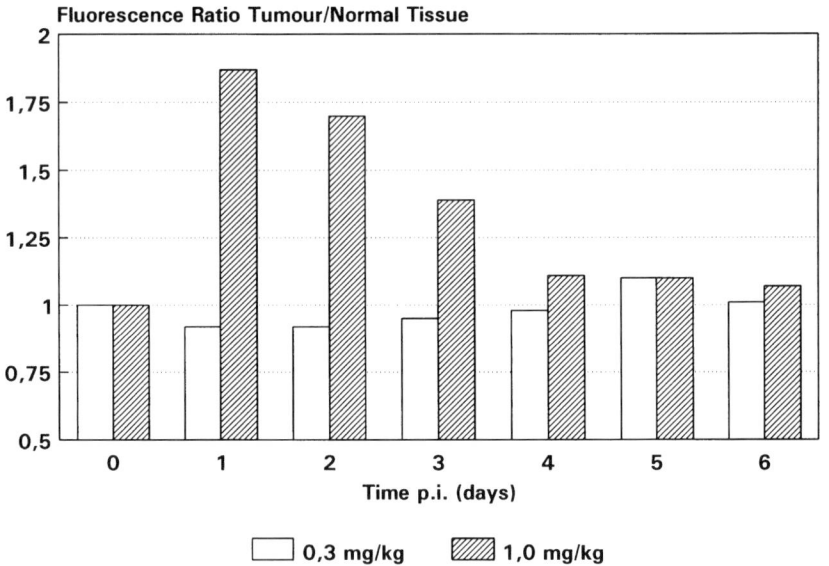

Fig. 9.4. Ratio of tumour to normal tissue fluorescence in the observation chamber model as a function of time after injection of 0.3 mg/kg *m*-THPC (*n* =9) and 1 mg/kg *m*-THPC (*n*=4, as in Fig. 9.3.). The fluorescence ratios after 0.3 mg/kg were not significantly different from the (auto)fluorescence ratio before drug injection. There was a slight increase in the 'absolute' fluorescence values at day one but this was not much more than 10% above the autofluorescence.

Photodynamic therapy

Photodynamic therapy with HpD or Photofrin causes immediate and strong vascular effects (Star et al 1986). The earliest phenomenon is ischaemia. The normal arterioles and the blood vessels in the tumour practically 'disappear'. To a lesser extent this also occurs in the normal capillaries. The larger venules show vasoconstriction. Ischaemia at the end of irradiation is often followed by partial or complete reperfusion, but the circulation is then slow and eventually a partial or complete vascular stasis results, depending on the drug/light dose combination. Haemorrhage may occur in the tumour and to a lesser extent in the normal tissue (capillaries) also depending on the drug/light dose combination. Often platelet aggregates are seen adhering to the blood vessel wall, temporarily blocking the circulation and being carried away by the blood circulation later. Comparing Figure 9.5 A2 with Fig. 9.5 A1 the ischaemia in the tumour is just discernable and the blood vessels around the tumour appear constricted. This is more pronounced at the end of the irradiation in Figure 9.5 A3, but then tumour vessels show reperfusion, partial stasis and focal haemorrhage.

PDT with *m*-THPC caused a less pronounced immediate vascular reponse. Figures 9.5 B1–B3 show little difference except for minor vasoconstriction observable in Figure 9.5 B3. Immediately after irradiation the blood vessels and the circulation in tumour and normal tissue appeared normal. The irradiation time was short (3.3 min) but for the same final response (see Fig. 9.6) PDT with HpD/Photofrin results in more pronounced acute effects, also for short treatment times. In particular, ischaemia of the tumour occurs during irradiation in PDT with HpD but not in PDT with *m*-THPC. Two hours after irradiation (Fig. 9.5 B3, 0.3 mg/kg *m*-THPC and PDT 1 d p.i.) 50% stasis was seen in the tumour and slightly reduced circulation in the subcutaneous tissue. One day later the tumour was necrotic and the normal tissue showed a partial stop of circulation (mean score 6 in Fig. 9.6 B, III). With a dose of 1.0 mg/kg *m*-THPC and irradiation`3 days p.i. the vascular effects immediately after irradiation were still minor. Two hours later there was partial stasis in the tumour with some haemorrhage. One day later the tumour was necrotic and the normal tissue showed complete vascular stasis. Even though the vascular response in *m*-THPC-PDT was delayed compared to HpD-PDT, tumour and normal tissue necrosis was always associated with vascular stasis. Tumour regrowth in this model was only prevented when the tumour and a margin of the surrounding normal tissue became necrotic after PDT. In this respect, no difference was seen between *m*-THPC mediated PDT and HpD-PDT or Photofrin-PDT.

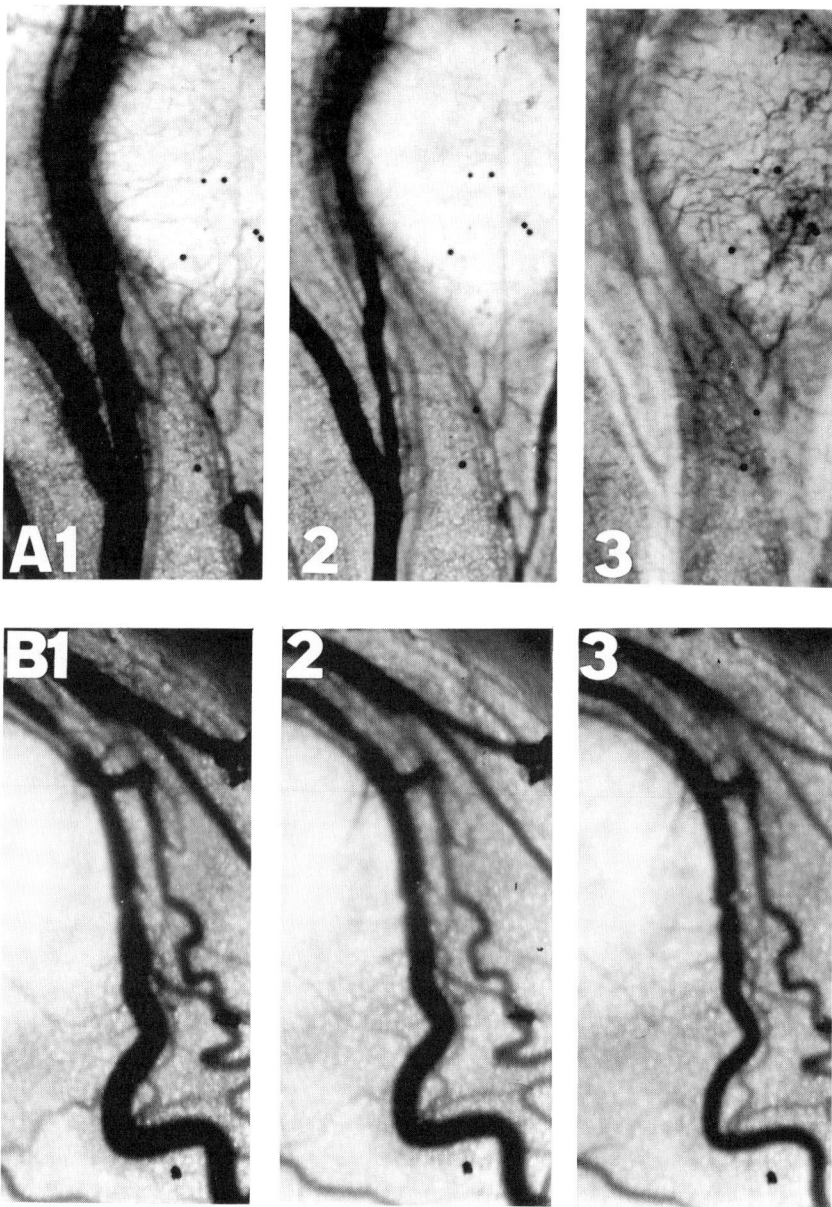

Fig. 9.5. Comparison of vascular effects during and after PDT with HpD and with *m*-THPC. A1–A3: HpD, 15 mg/kg, irradiation 24 h p.i. at 60 mW/cm² during 50 min (180 J/cm², 630 nm). The tumour is in the upper right of the photographs. B1–B3: *m*-THPC, 0.3 mg/kg, irradiated 24 h p.i. at 50 mW/cm² during 3.3 minutes (10 J/cm², 652 nm). The tumour is the light area to the left of the large venule. A1: Before irradiation; A2: after 10 min of irradiation (36 J/cm²); A3: At the end of irradiation (50 min). B1: Before irradiation; B2: at the end of irradiation (3.3 min); B3: 2 h after irradiation.

DISCUSSION

This paper does not describe a completed study, but should be considered as a report on work in progress. Some of the reported phenomena have been observed with only a small number of animals and should therefore be regarded with some caution. Nevertheless, the differences noted between fluorescence and PDT with HpD/Photofrin and *m*-THPC are so pronounced that they are not likely to change considerably when the number of animals is increased. With these considerations in mind we present the following discussion.

Fluorescence

Based on fluorescence, HpD and Photofrin are not particularly good tumour localizers in our model. Nevertheless, tumours in animals and humans have shown selective fluorescence with these drugs (Baumgartner et al 1987, Lam et al 1990, Unsöld et al 1990). However, we use a tumour transplanted in skin tissue, a normal tissue which tends to retain haematoporphyrin derivatives. In the reports referred to above the tumours were located in mucosa. Futhermore, the fluorescent components of HpD/Photofrin are probably monomers, whereas the components responsible for the photodynamic activity are most likely dimers and oligomers which show little fluorescence. In this respect *m*-THPC is a better drug, because it is a single compound so that fluorescence and photodynamic activity are mediated by the same substance. Nevertheless, there is no clear relationship between fluorescence and PDT-effects using *m*-THPC (discussion below).

   m-THPC is a remarkably good tumour localizer in our model. The fact that at any fluorescence measured in the blood vessels was weak compared to the maximum tumour fluorescence suggests an active accumulation process. It is also possible that some chemical modification or binding occurs which changes the fluorescence and/or photodynamic properties of *m*-THPC. Maximum tumour fluorescence following 1 mg/kg i.v. was observed 3 days p.i. and the optimum tumour/normal tissue ratio occurred 1 day p.i. These are long intervals compared to other drugs studied in our model. For example, the optimum interval for $AlPcS_4$, the best tumour localizer of the sulphonated Al- and Zn-phthalocyanines, is 30–60 min. p.i. (Van Leengoed et al 1993). We note that selectivity appears to result from the fact that the drug accumulates more quickly in the tumour than in the normal tissue. The normal tissue is seen to eventually 'catch up' causing the tumour normal tissue fluorescence ratio to diminish. This pattern is seen with most drugs studied in our model, with a different time scale for each drug. Selective tumour fluorescence appears to depend on *m*-THPC concentration (Figs 9.3 and 9.4). The number of animals in the fluorescence study makes it highly unlikely that this drug dose effect is due to random variations. In the same concentration range Bonnet et al (1989) have observed a rapid change in depth of tumour necrosis following PDT. This phenomenon requires further study. If for clinical applications the drug dose must be reduced to minimize induced skin photosensitivity and if this would adversely affect the selective uptake/retention of m-THPC in tumour tissue, this drug would lose one attractive property. However, it might still be attractive because of its high photodynamic activity, provided the latter would decrease less rapidly than the fluorescence upon reducing the drug dose.

Photodynamic therapy

m-THPC is a highly effective drug for PDT. This is of particular practical importance, because with available lasers it is often a problem to deliver in a reasonable time the light dose required in clinical PDT. An outstanding example is the treatment of mesothelioma by PDT (Ris et al 1991).

We have observed circulation damage in PDT with m-THPC. The acute vascular effects were much less pronounced than with HpD or Photofrin-mediated PDT. If this would mean that the tissue oxygenation remains intact during irradiation, increased direct tumour cell killing might be possible, depending on where the drug is accumulated (e.g. tumour cells, endothelial cells). The observation chamber model does not provide information on the relative importance of direct tumour cell killing versus secondary tumour cell death resulting from vascular stasis.

Despite weak and non-selective tumour fluorescence one day after 0.3 mg/kg m-THPC i.v. (Fig. 9.4), irradiation with 10 J/cm^2 yielded complete vascular stasis in the tumour and partial stasis in the normal tissue (Fig. 9.6). A partial explanation could be that tumour blood vessels (capillaries) are weaker and more easily damaged than normal tissue blood vessels. In this context it should be noted that Ris et al (1993) measured a much larger depth of necrosis in tumour tissue than in normal tissue, even though the m-THPC concentration in tumour tissues was only slightly larger than in normal tissue.

Increasing the interval between m-THPC-injection (0.3 mg/kg) and irradiation from 1 day to 3 days caused a considerable reduction in PDT-induced vascular damage (Fig. 9.6). Ris et al (1993), on the other hand, found little reduction in depth of tumour and normal tissue necrosis in mice for the same m-THPC dose and the same intervals.

With 1.0 mg/kg m-THPC irradiation was performed 3 days p.i. at the tumour fluorescence maximum. The light dose of 10 J/cm^2 was apparently large enough to cause complete and non-selective stasis of tumour and normal tissue circulation. It would be interesting to see whether irradiating at the interval of maximum selectivity and reducing the light dose would make it possible to achieve selective tumour necrosis in the observation chamber model.

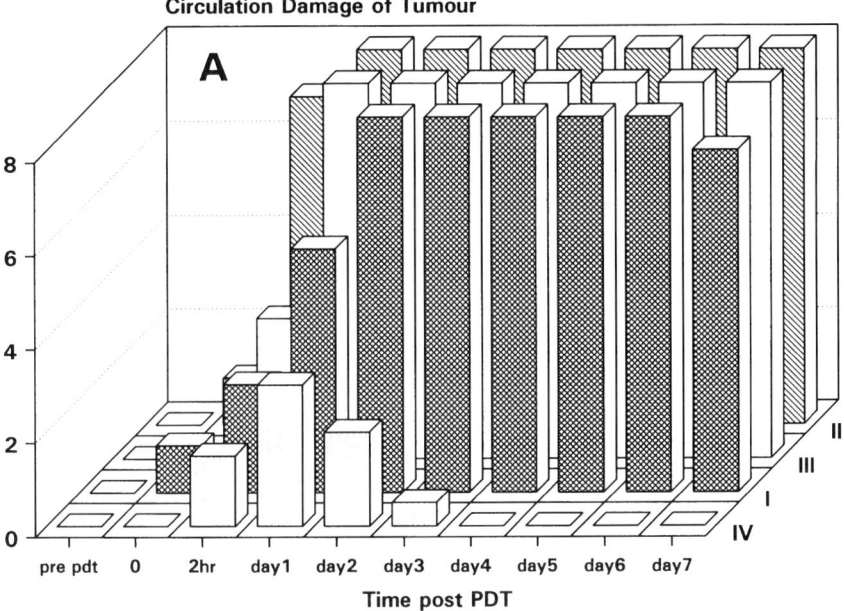

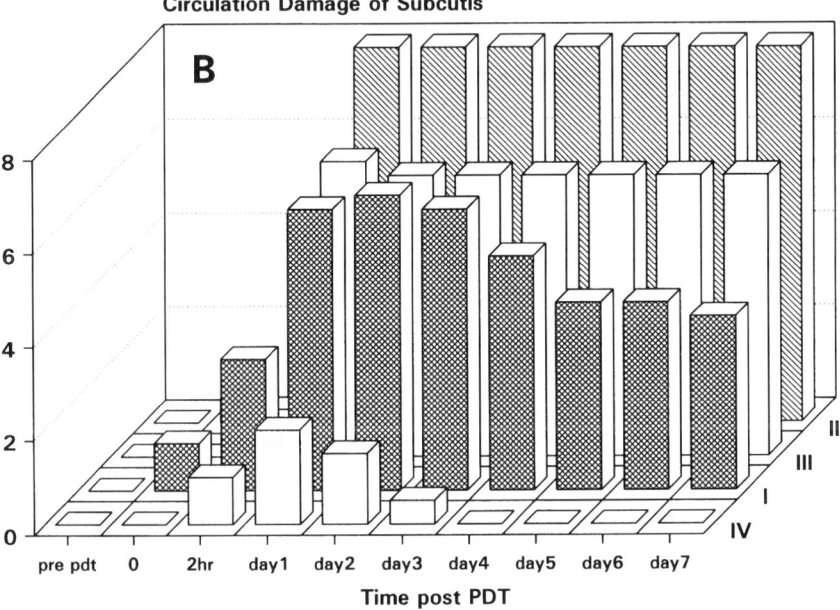

Fig. 9.6. Effects on the blood circulation in tumour (A) and normal tissue (B) caused by PDT with Photofrin and with *m*-THPC, as a function of time after treatment. The bars at day 0 indicate the score immediately after irradiation. I: Photofrin, 10 mg/kg, irradiated 24 h p.i. with 25 J/cm² (4.17 min, 625 nm, *n*=3); II: *m*-THPC, 1.0 mg/kg, irradiated 72 h p.i. with 10 J/cm² at 50 mW/cm² (3.3 min, 652 nm, *n*=2); III: *m*-THPC, 0.3 mg/kg, irradiated 24 h p.i. with 10 J/cm² (*n*=3); IV: *m*-THPC, 0.3 mg/kg, irradiated 72 h p.i. with 10 J/cm² (*n*=2).

REFERENCES

Baumgartner R, Fisslinger H, Jocham D, Lenz H, Ruprecht L, Stepp H, Unsöld E 1987 A fluorescence imaging device for endoscopic detection of early stage cancer – instrumental and experimental studies. Photochemistry and Photobiology 46: 759–763

Bonnet R, White RD, Winfield U-J, Berenbaum MC 1989 Hydroporphyrins of the *meta*-tetra(hydroxyphenyl)porphyrin series as tumour photosensitizers. Biochemical Journal 261: 277–280

Dougherty TJ, Marcus SL (1992) Photodynamic therapy. European Journal of Cancer 28A: 1734–1742

Lam S, Palcic B, McLean D, Hung J, Korbelik M, Profio EA (1990) Detection of early lung cancer using low dose photofrin II. Chest 97: 333–337

Reinhold HS, Blachiewics B, Van den Berg-Blok AE (1981) Reoxygenation of tumors in 'sandwich' chambers. European Journal of Cancer and Clinical Oncology 17: 781–795

Ris H-B, Altermatt HJ, Inderbitzi R, Hess R, Nachbur B, Stewart JCM, Wang Q, Lim CK, Bonnet R, Berenbaum MC, Althaus U (1991) Photodynamic therapy with chlorins for diffuse malignant mesothelioma: initial clinical results. British Journal of Cancer 64: 1116–1120

Ris H-B, Altermatt HJ, Nachbur B, Stewart JCM, Wang Q, Lim CK, Bonnet R, Althaus U (1993) Effect of drug-light interval on photodynamic therapy with *meta*-tetrahydroxyphenylchlorin in malignant mesothelioma. International Journal of Cancer 53: 141–146

Star WM, Marijnissen JPA, Van den Berg-Blok AE, Versteeg AAC, Franken NAP, Reinhold HS (1986) Destruction of rat mammary tumor and normal tissue microcirculation by hematoporphyrin derivative photoradiation observed in vivo in sandwich observation chambers. Cancer Research 46: 2532–2540

Star W, Versteeg J, Van Putten W, Marijnissen H (1990) Wavelength dependence of hematoporphyrin derivative photodynamic treatment effects on rat ears. Photochemistry and Photobiology 52: 547–554

Unsöld E, Baumgartner R, Beyer W, Jocham D, Stepp H (1990). Fluorescence detection and photodynamic treatment of photosensitized tumours in special consideratrion of urology. Lasers in Medical Science 5: 207–212

Van Leengoed E, Versteeg J, Van der Veen N, Van den Berg-Blok A, Marijnissen H, Star W (1990) Tissue-localizing properties of some photosensitizers studied by in vivo fluorescence imaging. Journal of Photochemistry and Photobiology B: Biology 6: 111–119

Van Leengoed HLLM, Van der Veen N, Versteeg AAC, Ouellet R, Van Lier JE, Star WM (1993) In vivo fluorescence kinetics of phthalocyanines in a skin fold observation chamber model: role of central metal ion and degree of sulphonation. Photochemistry and Photobiology 58: 233–237

10. A standardized methodology for evaluation of photoactive anti-tumour agents as applied to *meta*-tetra(hydroxyphenyl)-chlorin

L. A. Lofgren   A. M. Ronn   A. L. Abramson
M. J. Shikowitz   M. Nouri   B. M. Steinberg

INTRODUCTION

Photodynamic therapy (PDT), used either as a primary or adjunctive treatment for benign and malignant tumours, is of great interest. This therapy is based on activation of a chemical by visible light, resulting in a cascade of events that eventually results in the destruction of the tumour. The drugs used for PDT have three specific characteristics. First, they absorb light in the visible wavelengths. Second, they transfer the absorbed energy to ambient triplet, resulting in the formation of singlet oxygen, which is highly toxic to cells. Finally, they show selectivity, i.e. they are preferentially retained in some tissues longer than others. PDT has been used clinically with good results (Marcus 1990, Kato 1990). However, a major limitation on this therapy for ambulatory patients has been the prolonged photosensitivity of the skin, due to retention of drug (Mullooly et al 1990).

In order to evaluate and compare new photosensitizers, and establish the parameters for clinical trials, it is necessary to establish a model system that permits evaluation of all parameters of PDT. These include minimal toxicity in the absence of light, selectivity for tumour tissue, high energy yield when activated by light resulting in specific destruction of the tumour with minimal or no damage to the surrounding normal tissue, and good light penetration of tissue. This can be done in a multitude of ways, but there is no standard procedure currently in use.

We describe a structured and methodical approach by which any drug with promising chemical properties (stable composition, absorption in the red portion of the spectrum to facilitate penetration) and minimal general toxicity in preliminary studies, can be evaluated for therapeutic usefulness.

Our standardized protocol evaluates three key parameters. Selectivity in tumours is measured by a relative retention ratio (triple R). Safety is measured by tissue tolerance to treatment (triple T) parameters. This test also provides a method by which photosensitizers can be compared to each other for biological standardization. Efficacy is measured by disappearance of tumours and by possible recurrence during a protracted follow-up period.

The studies are based on a tumour model we used originally for studies with HPD (Shikowitz et al 1986): cutaneous papillomas on rabbits, induced by cottontail rabbit papillomavirus (CRPV). This model has the advantages that the tumour grows in a matrix of normal tissue of the same type, that multiple tumours can be established on a single animal, that the tumours do not endanger the health of the animal during prolonged follow up, and that the benign tumours exhibit the highly vascularized histology characteristic of malignant tumors.

The application of this approach is illustrated with our studies of meta-tetra(hydroxyphenyl)chlorin (m-THPC) (Lofgren et al 1994), a sensitizer originally described by Bonnett et al (1989). Berenbaum et al (1986) have reported that m-THPC is highly potent, causing significant tumour necrosis in rodents at dose levels where the corresponding porphyrins are not effective. Clinically, m-THPC has been used for the treatment of diffuse malignant mesothelioma with promising results (Ris et al 1991). Our studies have supported the earlier observations, and established the parameters for application of this photosensitizer to other types of tumors.

MATERIALS AND METHODS

Rabbits and virus inoculations

Dutch Belted and New Zealand White Rabbits were inoculated with CRPV and used for studies of relative retention, tissue tolerance and efficacy (Lofgren et al 1994). The technique used for inoculation was a modification of the technique previously described by Shikowitz et al (1986). Briefly, the rabbits were shaved and each site for inoculation tattooed with four dots, marking the corners of a 1 cm square. A drop of crude CRPV suspension was placed on the skin in the center of the tattooed square and a professional tattoo needle lightly jabbed by hand 20 times through the drop. After 6 to 12 weeks, papillomas with a base diameter of 5 to 30 mm had developed in the inoculated areas.

Photosensitizer and light

m-THPC is a synthesized chemical, obtained from Scotia Pharmaceuticals Ltd (Guildford, Surrey, England). The formulation used in our study (Batch PK23K) was composed of 91.7% m-THPC, 5.9% meta-tetra (hydroxyphenyl)porphyrin, and 2.4% hydroxylated derivatives of m-THPC. The drug, supplied as a sterile lyophilized powder, was dissolved in a mixture of polyethylene glycol 400 and ethanol to a final concentration of 4 mg/ml. The drug dose used in all studies (with one exception, see below) was 0.3 mg/kg body weight, the same dose used in treatments of humans (Ris et al 1991).

Light was generated by an argon ion laser emitting at 652 nm. A 400 μm diameter quartz fibre with a straight microlens fibre was attached via a fibre coupler. Irradiance was kept at 100 mW/cm^2 except where noted.

A 33-gauge copper-constantan miniature hypodermic thermocouple probe was inserted under the rabbit skin in the areas given the highest light dose, connected to a thermometer to determine elevation of temperature during PDT. Sensitivity of measurement was 0.10°C. Elevation in skin temperatures during exposure did not exceed 1.5°C.

Drug concentration measurements

Blood samples were collected and several 10 to 30 mg biopsies were taken from papillomas and skin at time points ranging from minutes to 4 weeks after injection of *m*-THPC. Tissues were frozen in liquid nitrogen and pulverized in a Teflon chamber with a steel ball, using a Braun Micro Dismembrator II. Dimethyl sulphoxide, 1 ml, was added to every 10 mg of tissue which was rotated on a wheel for 1 h, and the suspension centrifuged at 15 000 r.p.m. The supernatant was excited at 420 nm in a Shimadzu RF-540 spectrofluorophotometer with an emission range of 600 to 700 nm. The height of the 652 nm peak was compared to an *m*-THPC standard provided by Scotia Pharmaceuticals Ltd. This technique permitted an analysis of up to 40 samples per day. The lowest detectable concentration with a reliable signal-to-noise ratio was 40 pg/g tissue.

Triple T test

Various intervals between drug injection and exposure of the skin were evaluated. Rabbits were shaved on the back as described earlier. A masking device was made from aluminum foil and double-sided tape with a 1 cm circular hole. Exposed skin areas were examined and photographed at least every other day during the first week, and then at longer intervals depending on the reaction. Skin reactions were scored as follows:

1. No damage. Slight redness was permitted, but with no swelling or scarring at any time point.
2. Slight damage. Swelling of skin with or without blanching or redness. Barely visible scar permitted. Intradermal petechial bleeding may occur. Loss of tissue in exposed area with intact epithelium is accepted (depression in exposed area).
3. Moderate damage. Destruction of skin but not full thickness, resulting in a superficial scar.

4. Severe damage, indicated initially by chalk-white skin or blue-grey skin, resulting in thick eschar formation or deep ulceration. These lesions healed with a barely noticeable scar within 3 months, and usually much sooner.

Efficacy studies

These studies used rabbits with well-established warts. Each rabbit had multiple warts, and each wart on a rabbit was exposed to a different light dose, so that the set received all of the light doses tested. One additional papilloma on each rabbit was not exposed to light, as a control to exclude regression due to immunological response to the papillomas during the 3 month follow-up. Blood samples were taken at the time of treatment to measure m-THPC concentration. Normal skin surrounding the papillomas was masked with the aluminum foil, but a minimum 5 mm ring of normal skin surrounding the papilloma was always exposed to evaluate the reaction of normal tissue.

Rabbits were examined weekly and results documented with colour photographs labelled with date, treatment data and a millimetre scale. Final results were determined after a follow-up of 3 months. Complete response (CR) was defined as total regression of the papilloma. Partial response (PR) was defined as a decrease in wart area of greater than 50% with a final thickness of more than 3 mm, or a reduction in area of just less than 50% with a thickness of less than 3 mm. A decrease in size of less than 50% with a final thickness of greater than 3 mm was defined as no response (NR).

RESULTS

Triple R test

Before evaluating the efficacy of PDT for tumour treatment, it is necessary to determine the optimal interval between drug injection and treatment, and the maximum light dose that will not damage normal tissue adjacent to the tumour. Our first aim was therefore to conduct triple R tests, measuring drug in normal and papilloma tissue and in plasma at varying times after injection of m-THPC. The time point with the highest tumour:normal tissue ratio would be expected to be optimal for therapy.

m-THPC levels in plasma, papilloma and skin at different intervals after injection of drug are shown in Table 10.1. The highest ratio of m-THPC concentration in papilloma compared to normal skin was achieved at approximately 3 to 4 days, and was maintained until 8 d after injection. These results suggested that the optimum time for therapy would be during this interval. Initially, the plasma concentration was high, but after the first day it was lower than the concentration in papilloma and skin.

These studies were done with the drug dose previously used by Berenbaum et al (1986) and Ris et al (1991). If that data had not been available, it would have been necessary to repeat the studies with additional drug doses.

Table 10.1   Retention of *m*-THPC in normal and wart tissues and plasma

| Days | Extrapolated *m*-THPC concentration (ng/g) | | |
	Papilloma	Skin	Plasma
0.04	40	12	154
2	110	70	25
4	107	14	8
6	104	10	8
8	100	10	5
10	90	12	3
12	75	12	0
14	55	12	—
21	6	0	—

Adapted from Lofgren et al (1994).

Triple T test

Next, we evaluated the triple T parameters. This is the maximum light dose that can be applied to normal tissue after injection of a photosensitizer without causing permanent damage, at a time of maximum theoretical relative retention in tumour. Multiple parameters can be altered in this test, changing the biological effects of light exposure. To determine these parameters, we established 'skin ladders', testing the effects of increasing light doses as a function of drug dose with washout times ranging from 6 h to 28 d. Skin exposures of 10, 20, 40 and 80 J/cm² were routinely carried out, using only the areas of white skin on the Dutch belted rabbits. Additional bracketing doses were used occasionally, with 5 and 320 J/cm² as the lowest and highest doses.

Even a very low light dose (5 J/cm²) caused a severe skin reaction when the interval between injection and exposure was short (6 h), though we used the standard drug dose of 0.3 mg/kg. At this time the plasma concentrations were high. With a drug dose of 0.9 mg/kg and a moderate washout time, 25 J/cm² caused a severe reaction. In contrast, very long intervals (19–28 days) caused only a slight swelling of the skin with a light dose of 100 J/cm², and a dose of 40 J/cm² gave no reaction. The relationship between light dose and skin response at varying times after injection of 0.3 mg/kg is shown in Figure 10.1. This data clearly shows the interaction between these different parameters.

Interestingly, no more than slight skin damage could be achieved with any light dose up to and including 320 J/cm^2 in New Zealand White rabbits given the standard m-THPC dose of 0.3 mg/kg. Severe damage was achieved only after increasing the drug dose to 0.9 mg/kg.

Efficacy studies

The results described above defined the parameters for efficacy studies, using 0.3 mg/kg m-THPC and irradiating at 6 d post-injection with light doses ranging from 25 to 75 J/cm^2. The goal of this part of the study was to determine whether PDT of the tumours would be effective at light doses and a washout time that did not cause excessive damage to surrounding normal tissue.

Three parameters affected efficacy: light dose, effective drug dose and size of the warts (Table 10.2). Using a light dose of 50 J/cm^2, 40% of papillomas were cured, and another 40% showed partial response. When the light dose was increased to 75 J/cm^2, all papillomas showed either

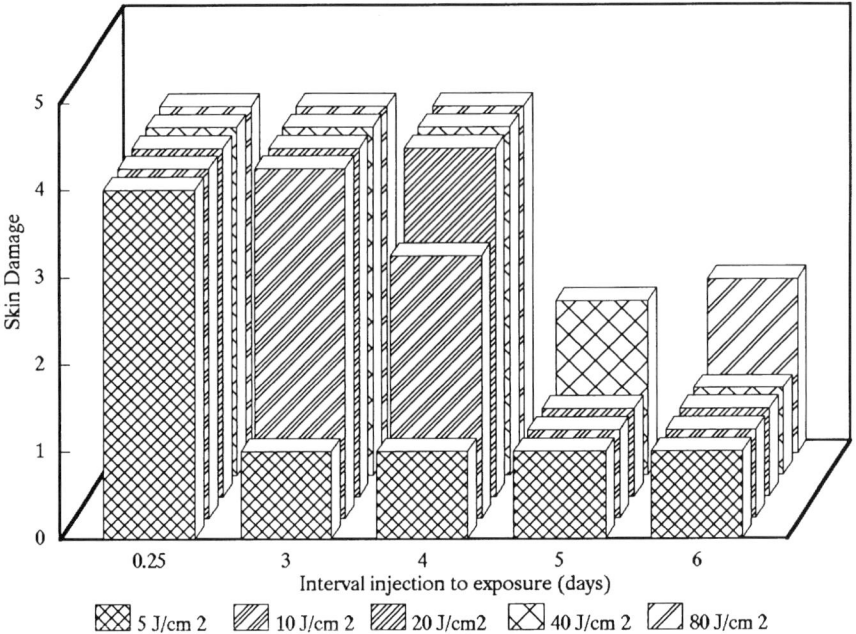

Fig. 10.1   Effects of varying light dose on skin response at varying times after injection of m-THPC. 1: no damage; 2: slight damage; 3: moderate damage; 4: severe damage. (Adapted from Lofgren et al 1994.)

complete or partial response, with a cure rate of 66%. There was no damage to the normal surrounding tissue. This is in contrast to DHE, where an equivalent light dose for therapy caused necrosis of the surrounding normal tissue. This also reflects the improved papilloma localization of this drug (*m*-THPC 10:1, DHE 2:1).

Table 10.2   Efficacy of *m*-THPC phototherapy

Effect	Light dose (J/cm2)			Plasma concentration		Papilloma size		
	25	50	75	Low	High	Small	Med.	Large
NR	2/5	1/5	0/6	2/6	1/10	1/4	0/4	2/8
PR	1/5	2/5	2/6	3/6	2/10	0/4	1/4	4/8
CR	2/5	2/5	4/6	1/6	7/10	3/4	3/4	2/8

Responses were scored as follows. NR: no response, or reduction in wart size of less than 50%, with a final thickness of greater than 3 mm. PR: partial response with reduction greater than NR, but with continued persistence. CR: complete response, with total regression of the wart and no recurrence during a three month follow up. The table shows the number of warts with each response divided by the number treated. Modified from Lofgren et al (1994).

Even though all animals were injected with the same drug dose, not all had the same circulating plasma levels at the time of treatment. Those animals with higher plasma levels (> 9.5 ng/ml) had 70% cure rates, with an additional 20% of warts showing partial response. In contrast, only 16% of warts showed complete remission if the circulating plasma levels were less than 5.5 ng/ml.

Finally, the size of the wart being treated (less than 50 mm^2, 50 to 100 mm^2, and greater than 100 mm^2) also affected response. This probably reflects limitations of light penetration to the base of highly keratinized large warts.

DISCUSSION

There has recently been a great deal of interest in new photosensitizers. We have described a methodology for the evaluation of any of these new photosensitizers prior to clinical studies. The structure of the photosensitizer determines its activities, and in part this can be predicted. Depth of light penetration steeply increases in soft tissue between 600–650 nm (Wilson & Patterson 1990), and absorption of red light can be enhanced by reducing the porphyrin molecule to the chlorin (Selman et al 1987, Kessel & Smith 1989). *m*-THPC, the drug we have studied, has an increased absorption of red light at 650 nm, resulting in increased tumour and tissue penetration. Berenbaum et al (1986) studied the tetra(hydroxyphenyl)porphyrins and found them on a molar basis to be about 25 times as potent as HPD in sensitizing subcutaneous tumours, and Bonnet et al

(1989), using a rodent model, found *m*-THPC considerably more potent as a tumour photosensitizer than the tetra(hydroxyphenyl)porphyrins. However, ideal photosensitizers for PDT cannot be predicted based only on such physical features.

The single most important feature of photodynamic therapy is the selective retention of drug in tumour compared to normal surrounding tissue. Unfortunately, the drugs in current use, and even most of the new drugs being investigated, have a rather small differential retention (Tralau et al 1990). Determination of this property is critical. However, selective retention cannot be directly used to predict clinical efficacy or tissue sensitivity. Variations in many factors can influence both clinical efficacy and safety parameters. An example of this dichotomy is our finding of a difference between the two strains of rabbits. There was no difference between the drug concentrations in the skin of Dutch Belted and New Zealand White rabbits, or between the tumour/skin ratios, but there was a significant difference in the reaction of normal skin to the same dose of light. Incremented skin damage (the skin ladder) could only be achieved with increasing light dose if the drug dose were significantly elevated. Thus clinical studies should always include individuals from different geographical regions and different races, since such variations in response cannot be predicted.

Animal experiments with photosensitizers often do not provide a rationale for choice of drug dose. The doses are frequently significantly higher than the corresponding human dose (Jefferis et al 1991), which can cause indiscriminate, undesirable destruction of tissue. We propose that a drug dose should be chosen by combining information on its triple R ratio and the triple T tests. Preferably, this testing should be done in a model system with a tumour surrounded by its normal tissue counterpart, and with studies of tissues corresponding to the intended clinical situation.

We chose our triple T scoring system to cover multiple time points after exposure to more than one drug dose, and to include a superficial destruction of normal skin. The aim of this testing was to determine a light dose for treatment of tumours below the threshold for normal tissue damage. The intermediate reactions of slight and moderate damage are subjective but we believe that they are necessary to describe the incremental skin lesions. This approach, if used at time of therapy, also provides a check that the exposures have been carried out correctly.

An unexpected finding was the marked impact of *m*-THPC plasma concentration on treatment efficacy (Table 10.2). Our hypothesis was that plasma levels would not be significant once the plasma curve approached baseline, which it does before day 6 after injection, while the concentration in papillomas is still high (Table 10.1). Based on this result, we suggest that it might be worthwhile to measure plasma levels of any drug in patients on the day of treatment and possibly adjust the light dose.

ACKNOWLEDGEMENTS

This work was supported by grant P50 DC – 00203 from the National Institute for Deafness and Other Communication Disorders, and grants from the Irving and Helen Schneider family, the Morris S. and Florence H. Bender foundation, the Otolaryngology foundation, the Swedish Cancer foundation (2809-B91-02XAB, 03XBB, 01PAC, 02PBC and 03PCC) and Örebro Medical Centre Hospital, Örebro, Sweden.

REFERENCES

Berenbaum MC, Akande SL, Bonnett R, et al 1986 meso-tetra(hydroxyphenyl)porphyrins, a new class of potent tumour photosensitizers with favorable selectivity. British Journal of Cancer 54: 717–725

Bonnett R, White RD, Winfield U-J, Berenbaum MC 1989 Hydroporphyrins of the meso-tetra(hydroxyphenyl)porphyrin series as tumor photosensitizers. Biochemical Journal 261: 277–280

Jefferis AF, Chevretton EB, Berenbaum MC 1991 Muscle damage and recovery in the rabbit tongue following photodynamic therapy with haematoporphyrin derivative. Acta Otolaryngologica (Stockholm) 111: 153–160

Kato H 1990 Photodynamic therapy of early cancers In: Morstyn G, Kaye A (eds) Phototherapy of cancer. Harwood Academic Publishers, Chur, Switzerland, pp 133–151

Kessel D, Smith K 1989 Photosensitization with derivatives of chlorophyll. Photochemistry and Photobiology 49: 157–160

Lofgren LA, Ronn AM, Abramson AL, Shikowitz MJ, Nouri M, Lee CJ, Batti J, Steinberg BM 1994 Photodynamic therapy using meso-tetra(hydroxyphenyl)chlorin: an animal model. Archives of Otolaryngology and Head and Neck Surgery in Press

Marcus SL (1990) Photodynamic therapy of human cancer: clinical status, potential and needs. In: Gomer CJ (ed) Future directions and applications in photodynamic therapy. SPIE Press, Bellingham, Washington, IS6: 5–56

Mullooly VM, Abramson AL, Shikowitz MJ (1990) Dihematoporphyrin ether-induced photosensitivity in laryngeal papilloma patients. Lasers in Surgery and Medicine 10: 349–356

Ris HB, Altermatt HJ, Inderbitzi R, et al 1991 Photodynamic therapy with chlorins for diffuse malignant mesothelioma: initial clinical results. British Journal of Cancer 64: 1116–1120

Selman SH, Garbo GM, Keck RW, Kreimer-Birnbaum M, Morgan AR 1987 A dose response analysis of purpurin derivatives used as photosensitizers for the photodynamic treatment of transplantable FANFT induced urothelial tumors. Journal of Urology 137: 1255–1257

Shikowitz MJ, Steinberg BM, Abramson AL 1986 Hematoporphyrin derivative therapy of papillomas – experimental Study. Archives of Otolaryngology and Head and Neck Surgery 112: 42–46

Tralau CJ, Barr H, MacRobert AJ, Bown SG 1990 Relative merits of porphyrins and pthalocyanine sensitization for photodynamic therapy, Vol 1. In: Kessel D (ed) Photodynamic therapy of neoplastic disease. CRC Press, Boca Raton, FL, pp 263–275

Wilson BC, Patterson MS 1990 The determination of light fluence distribution in photodynamic therapy. In: Kessel D, ed. Photodynamic therapy of neoplastic disease, Vol 1. CRC Press, Boston, MA, pp 129–145

11. Treatment effects of *meta*-tetra-(hydroxyphenyl)chlorin on the larynx

*A. L. Abramson L. A. Lofgren A. M. Ronn M. Nouri
B. M. Steinberg*

INTRODUCTION

Haematoporphyrin derivative (HPD) is a powerful photosensitizing agent that can cause destruction and death of tissues in which it has localized when activated by light of an appropriate wavelength. Photodynamic therapy (PDT) for benign and malignant tumours is based on the ability of the drug to be retained preferentially and to produce microvascular damage and cytotoxic agents when activated by visible light. HPD and its partially purified successor Porfimer sodium (Photofrin) have significant drawbacks because they are incompletely defined mixtures which have only low tumour selectivity, and cause significant skin photosensitization.

Second generation photosensitizers should, ideally, possess the following characteristics: (1) lack of toxicity in the dark, (2) constant stable composition, (3) selective photosensitization of tumour tissue, (4) high-triplet state yield with triplet energy greater than 94 kJ/mol, the excitation energy for singlet oxygen production, (5) absorption in the red portion of the visible spectrum (Bonnett et al 1989).

Absorption of the light in the red can be increased by reducing the porphyrin to the chlorin, which allows for a deeper tumouricidal effect (Selman et al 1987, Kessel & Smith 1989). It has been experimentally demonstrated that *meta*-tetra(hydroxyphenyl)chlorin (*m*-THPC) is markedly more potent and causes significant tumour necrosis at dose levels at which the corresponding porphyrin is ineffective (Berenbaum et al 1986). *m*-THPC has shown excellent tumour eradication and tissue selectivity in rodents, requiring only 10 J/cm^2 to induce tumour necrosis of 6 mm depth and minimal skin sensitivity. Clinically *m*-THPC has been used for the treatment of diffuse malignant mesothelioma with interesting results (Ris et al 1991).

Lofgren et al (1994) found that the optimum ratio of *m*-THPC drug concentration in the rabbit papilloma as compared to plasma and the normal surrounding skin occurred 4–8 days after sensitization. Using this time interval, 0.3 mg/kg of *m*-THPC was intravenously injected into the dog and the biodistribution established. The tissues within the larynx had median tissue concentrations of 95-120 ng/g.

Before this new photosensitizing drug (*m*-THPC) can be used in the treatment of human laryngeal papilloma, an experimental model must be used to investigate its pathological effects. Abramson et al (1988) using the dog model, established the safety parameters for delivery of PDT-HPD to the larynx and the same system was used to evaluate *m*-THPC.

MATERIALS AND METHODS

Institutional guidelines regarding animal experimentation were followed. Six days before surgery, 0.3 mg/kg of *m*-THPC was intravenously injected into healthy mongrel dogs weighing 7 to 10 kg. Anaesthesia consisted of intravenous pentobarbital sodium (30 mg/kg). At surgery, the dogs were spontaneously breathing without an endotracheal tube and placed in the supine position. The head was stabilized, a laryngoscope with multiple-port channels passed through the mouth, and the endolarynx exposed.

With an alligator forceps, a 33-gauge copper-constantan miniature hypodermic thermocoupler probe was placed through the laryngoscope and inserted immediately below the epithelium of the vocal cord. The thermocouple was then connected to a thermometer (Omega Digital 450-ATT) and readings obtained to a sensitivity of 0.1°C.

A Spectra-Physics argon ion laser (model 2016-05S) pumping a Spectra-Physics (Model 375) tunable dye laser was used to achieve a red light output at 652 nm for activating the photosensitive compound. A 400 µm diameter quartz fibre with a 1.5 cm cylindrical diffuser tip was then attached to the laser via a fibre coupler. After fibre calibration was completed and recorded for each predetermined energy setting, the flexible quartz fibre was placed through the centre port channel of the laryngoscope and into position approximately in the middle of the glottic inlet and at the level of the vocal cords.

In accordance with our experimental scheme, different power densities were delivered to the larynx by varying power output and time of exposure. At 24 h after surgery, an overdose of pentobarbital sodium was intravenously administered in sufficient amounts to kill the dogs. A total laryngectomy including the upper trachea was immediately performed and the interior visualized via a posterior incision. Observations were recorded and graded on a scale of 4 arbitrary units (Fig. 11.1) as to the degree of oedema and erythema present in the supraglottic, glottic, and subglottic regions. Gross specimen photographs were taken (using a Nikon FE 2 camera, ringflash, and Kodachrome ASA 64 film) at f-8 and 35 cm. from the larynx. Histological specimens were obtained and analysed from selective regions of the larynx (Abramson et al 1988).

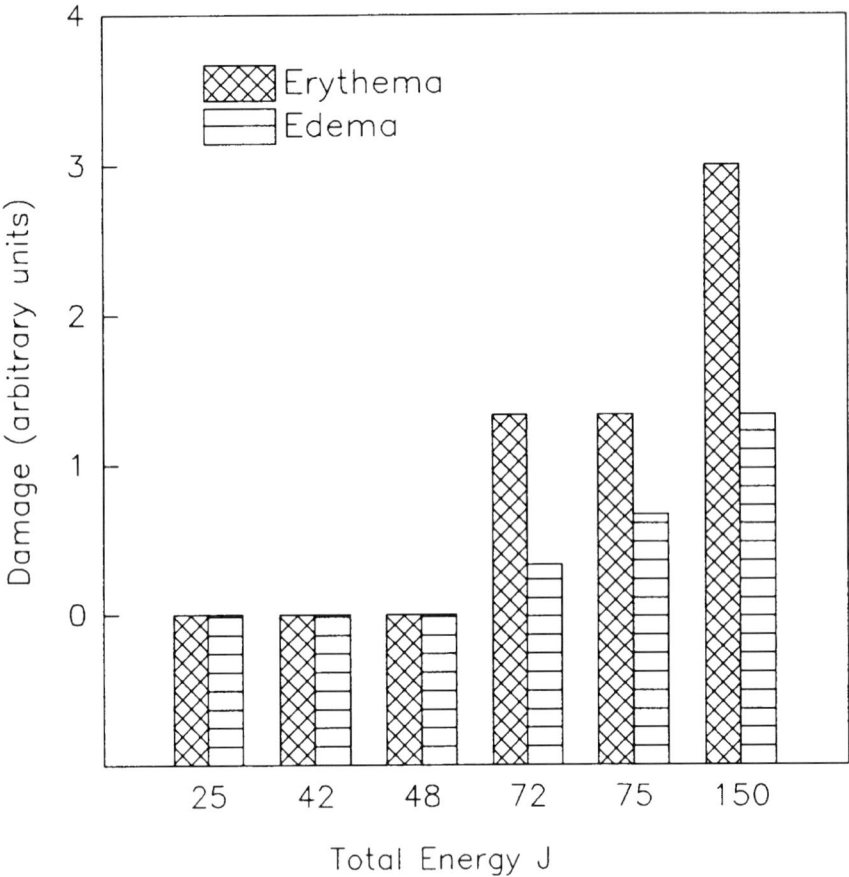

Fig. 11.1.   Oedema and erythema present in the supraglottic, glottic, and subglottic regions.

RESULTS

When increasing amounts of total energy were delivered to the canine larynx presensitized with *m*-THPC, progressive amounts of oedema and erythema were observed throughout the supraglottic, glottic, and subglottic
regions. On gross examination, there appeared to be three energy zones
that resulted in different grades of tissue response. Between 25 and 48 J
the larynx appeared normal except for minimal subglottic erythema. When
75 J was delivered, mild to moderate oedema and erythema were
observed. At 150 J severe oedema and moderate erythema were seen.
Prominent vascularity and erythema were most pronounced in the subglottic region. Significant oedema occurred within the lower supraglottic
region affecting the epiglottis, aryepiglottic folds, false cords, and vent-
ricle. However, oedema of the upper third of the epiglottis was lacking.

This area corresponded to where the laryngoscope had been placed when the red light was delivered.

The histological changes were dependent on the exposure energies. At 25 J alterations were minimal in the epithelium with some stasis changes in the small vessels. At 150 J, vascular changes were more pronounced, not only in the epithelium but in the submucosa. Oedema was seen in Reinkes space with associated inflammatory cells.

During PDT, the maximum change in temperature ranged from 0.3°C when 25 J was delivered to 1.9°C for 150 J.

DISCUSSION

The concept of using a photosensitive dye which is activated by light to selectively destroy tumour cells is not new (Tappeiner & Jesionek 1903).

Henderson et al (1980) induced squamous cell carcinomas on the shaved backs of white mice by repeated painting of a chemical carcinogen. Subsequently, after intraperitoneal injection of hematoporphyrin derivative, an intense red fluorescence was seen in the central tumour region. It was of interest that the chemically induced papillomas that were frequently present in the surrounding tissue also demonstrated a deep red fluorescence.

Experimentally, multiple large keratinized cutaneous papillomas were created on Dutch Belted rabbits using a cottontail rabbit papillomavirus (Shikowitz et al 1986). Following intravenous administration of HPD, PDT was given and marked regression and elimination of the papilloma was observed.

When various experimental tumours were heated within the range of 41°C, destruction occurred specifically in malignant cells without apparent damage to normal cells (Overgaard & Overgaard 1972). During this experiment a rise in temperature of the vocal cord (0.3°C to 1.9°C) was achieved after varying the amounts of total energy (25 to 150 J) delivered. Thus, the thermal effects that were generated within the larynx are alone insufficient to achieve a therapeutic response in either tumour tissue or destruction of normal laryngeal epithelium.

Using the canine model, safety parameters for delivery of PDT-HPD to the larynx were established. Between 10 and 40 J this organ appeared normal, with only mild erythema noted at 60 J. Above 100 J moderate to severe erythema and oedema were seen, with two upper-airway deaths observed (Abramson et al 1988).

With the above information, clinical treatment parameters for patients with recurrent laryngeal papillomatosis were established. It is important to note that just as our canine model had no significant pathological abnormalities when 50 J of energy was delivered, neither did our 35 patients with moderate to severe laryngeal papillomatosis (Abramson et al 1992). Thus for HPD type compounds the experimental animal model proved extremely useful in predicting the type of tissue response which occurred in the human larynx.

Berenbaum et al (1986) studied a new group of tumour sensitizers, the tetra(hydroxyphenyl)porphyrins. He found them on a molar basis to be about 25 times as potent as HPD in sensitizing subcutaneous tumours. Wilson & Patterson (1990) has shown that effective depth of penetration steeply increases in soft tissue between 600–650 nm (Feins et al 1990).

Absorption of light in the red can be enhanced by reducing the porphyrin to the chlorin (Selman et al 1987, Kessel & Smith 1989). *Meta*-tetra(hydroxyphenyl)chlorin has as expected an increased absorption of red light at 650 nm resulting in increased tumour and tissue penetrance.

Bonnett et al (1989) using a rodent model found *m*-THPC to be considerably more potent as a tumour photosensitizer then the tetra(hydroxyphenyl)porphyrins. Tumour photonecrosis within the chlorin group of chemicals was greatest with *m*-THPC requiring only 10 J/cm^2 to induce 6 mm of necrosis.

A nude mice model which had a malignant mesothelioma xenograft implant, was photosensitized with 0.3 mg *m*-THPC/kg and activated at 650 nm with 10 J/cm^2 (Feins et al 1990). It was found that the greatest therapeutic ratio between tumour normal tissue occurred when laser activation was performed 4 days after sensitization.

A clinical trial using *m*-THPC PDT was performed on patients with diffuse malignant mesothelioma (Ris et al 1991). It was found that when the interval between sensitization and activation was 48 h, 10 mm depth of tumour infarction was found and tissue concentration was up to 14 times higher in the tumour then in normal tissues. Skin photosensitivity was mild and occurred 3 to 10 days after photoactivation. One patient with chest wall recurrence of breast cancer was activated 9 days after *m*-THPC with 30 J/cm^2. The skin was spared while the underlying tumour disappeared.

Lofgren et al 1993 (unpublished observations) have described the biodistribution of *m*-THPC in a canine model. The drug concentration which was observed in the different organ systems was closely correlated with the capillary density.

In the larynx, the median tissue concentration (ng/g) of *m*-THPC was: cartilage (10), vocal cord muscle (95), vocal cord mucosa (105) and aryepiglottic fold (120). The highest concentration of *m*-THPC was found in the kidney (495).

In this experiment, the canine larynx model system was used. Increasing amounts of total energy (10 to 150 J) were delivered to the pre-sensitized (*m*-THPC) larynx. Very similar findings were observed when compared to HPD. It would appear that energy levels up to 50 J result in minimal pathological laryngeal changes with no significant erythema or edema.

ACKNOWLEDGEMENTS

This work was supported by Grant P50 DC 00203 from the National Institute for Deafness and Other Communication Disorders, the Irving and Helen Schneider Family and the Otolaryngology Foundation and by grants from the Swedish Cancer foundation (2809-B91-02XAB, 03XBB, 01PAC, 02PBC and 03PCC) and Örebro Medical Center Hospital, Sweden (L.A.L.).

REFERENCES

Abramson AL, Hirschfield LS, Shikowitz MJ, Barrezueta NX 1988 The pathologic effects of photodynamic therapy on the larynx. Archives of Otolaryngology and Head and Neck Surgery 114: 33–39

Abramson AL, Shikowitz MS, Mullooly VM et al 1992 Clinical effects of photodynamic therapy on recurrent laryngeal papillomas. Archives of Otolaryngology and Head and Neck Surgery 118: 25–29

Berenbaum MC, Akande SL, Bonnett R, Kaur H, Ioannou S, White RD 1986 Meso-tetra-(hydroxyphenyl)porphyrins, a new class of potent tumour photosensitizers with favourable selectivity. British Journal of Cancer 54: 712–725

Bonnett R, White RD, Winfield UJ, Berenbaum MC 1989 Hydroporphyrins of the meso-tetra(hydroxyphenyl)porphyrin series as tumour photosensitizers. Biochemical Journal 261: 277–280

Feins RH, Hilf R, Ross H, Gibson SL 1990 Photodynamic therapy for human malignant mesothelioma in the nude mouse. Journal of Surgical Research 49: 311

Henderson RW, Christie GS, Clezy PS, Lindman J 1980 Hematoporphyrin diacetate: a probe to distinguish malignant from normal tissue by selective fluorescence. British Journal of Experimental Pathology 61: 345–349

Kessel D, Smith K 1989 Photosensitization with derivatives of chlorophyll. Photochemistry and Photobiology 49: 157–160

Lofgren LA, Ronn AM, Abramson AL, Shikovitz MJ, Nouri M, Lee CJ, Batti J, Steinberg B 1994 Photodynamic therapy using meso-tetra(hydroxyphenyl)chlorin: an animal model. Archives of Otolaryngology and Head and Neck Surgery, in press.

Overgaard K, Overgaard J 1972 Investigations on the possibility of a thermic tumour therapy: I. Short-wave treatment of a transplanted isologous mouse mammary carcinoma. European Journal of Cancer and Clinical Oncology 8: 65–78.

Ris HB, Altermatt HJ, Inderbitzi R et al 1991 Photodynamic therapy with chlorins for diffuse malignant mesothelioma: initial clinical results. British Journal of Cancer 164: 1116–1120

Selman S H, Garbo G M, Keck R W, Kreimer-Birnbaum M, Morgan A R 1987 A dose response analysis of porphyrin derivatives used as photosensitizers for the photodynamic treatment of transplantable FANFI induced urothelial tumors. Journal of Urology 137: 1255–1257

Shikowitz M J, Steinberg B M, Abramson A L 1986 Hematoporphyrin derivative therapy of papillomas. Archives Otolaryngology and Head and Neck Surgery 112: 42–46

Tappeiner V H, Jesionek A 1903 Therapeutische Versuche mit Fluoreszierenden flouresceincended Stoffen. Munchener Mediciniscne Wochenschrift 50: 2042–2044

Wilson B C, Patterson M S 1990 The determination of light fluence distribution in photodynamic therapy. In: Kessel D ed. Photodynamic therapy of neoplastic disease Vol 1. CRC Press, Boston, p 129

12. Intra-operative photodynamic therapy with *meta*-tetra-(hydroxyphenyl)chlorin for chest malignancies

H. B. Ris H. J. Altermatt B. Nachbur J. C. M. Stewart
Q. Wang C. K. Lim R. Bonnett U. Althaus

INTRODUCTION

Photodynamic therapy (PDT) is an attractive antitumour therapy since it allows for selective tumour destruction while sparing unaffected tissues. It might be an useful adjunct to surgical tumour resection in situations without cleavage plane between tumour and underlying normal structures and for the treatment of tumours with a high tendency for local recurrence (despite correct resection). For thoracic malignancies this holds true for malignant mesothelioma, low grade sarcoma, malignant histiocytoma, intrathoracic metastases of malignant thymoma and some metastases of germ cell tumours. Several reports have documented the feasibility of intra-operative PDT after surgery under clinical conditions for retroperitoneal sarcomas[1], intraperitoneal tumor dissemination[2] and thoracic malignancies.[3,4] High tumour selectivity and efficacy for PDT is required in order to reduce treatment time and to spare underlying normal structures. Since haematoporphyrin derivative (HPD) is not an ideal sensitizer in this respect, new compounds are currently being developed. Among them, *meta*-tetra(hydroxyphenyl)chlorin (*m*-THPC) has shown excellent antitumour activity and tissue selectivity in rodents without causing significant toxicity.[5]

Since 1990 we have evaluated intraoperative PDT using *m*-THPC as sensitizer on selected patients with chest malignancies and the results are summarized in this report.

PATIENTS AND METHODS

Seven patients with malignant mesothelioma and one with recurrent malignant fibrous histiocytoma of the chest cavity underwent thoracotomy and surgical tumour resection followed by intra-operative *m*-THPC-PDT of the chest cavity involved. One patient was referred for recurrent breast cancer with extensive chest wall involvement and was treated by *m*-THPC-

PDT without surgery. PDT was performed as surface irradiance with non-thermal light doses on all nine patients. All patients understood the experimental design of this treatment and consent was obtained from the local Human Investigations Committee of our institution. Preliminary PDT was performed on two patients with mesothelioma at different drug–light conditions and drug–light intervals in order to optimize tumour ablation and to minimize damage to underlying vital structures. Tumour areas of 3 cm in diameter were treated at 650 nm, the light being delivered via thoracoscopy using a quartz optical fibre after i.v. administration of m/THPC. Biopsies were taken 5 d after light delivery and compared to untreated tumour.

From the results obtained, intra-operative *m*-THPC-PDT following tumour resection via thoracotomy was performed on eight patients. Four patients underwent extended pneumonectomy, two pleurectomy and lobectomy, and two decortication. The diaphragm was debulked yet pre-served in all patients in order to maintain this natural barrier against fur-ther tumour spread. All patients were given 0.3 mg *m*-THPC/kg i.v. and light was delivered at a drug–light interval of 48 h (four patients) and 72 h (four patients). After completion of the surgical procedure 10 J/cm² were applied through the open chest wound to the diaphragm and costophrenic sulcus in seven patients and 5 J/cm² to the remainder of the thoracic cavity in overlapping spots of about 7 cm diam in six patients.

The mediastinum was shielded by a moist towel if parts of the peri-cardium had to be removed (five patients). No irradiance of the upper tho-racic cavity and the upper lobe was performed on the patient with histiocytoma due to dense adhesions related to prior operations. One patient suffered from intractable pain due to tumour infiltration of the brachial plexus. Peritoneal tumour spread precluded major resection. Previous surgi-cal plexus release by a supraclavicular approach did not help to reduce the pain and *m*-THPC-PDT was performed to the plexus involved. The plexus was exposed through thoracotomy and local decortication of the pleural dome, and 10 J/cm², 0.1 W/cm² were delivered in overlapping spots of 2 cm diam by use of a lens, 72 h after administration of 0.3 mg *m*-THPC/kg.

One was patient was referred with recurrent breast cancer and extensive chest wall involvement. Since our experimental work on human tumour xenografts suggested that tumour selectivity of *m*-THPC-PDT might be considerably enhanced if, for a given drug dose, longer drug–light intervals are combined with higher light doses, this patient was treated accordingly. After i.v. application of 0.3 mg *m*-THPC/kg, tumour areas of 1.3 cm in diameter were treated by surface irradiance at drug–light intervals ranging from 4 to 9 days. The light dose applied was 10 J/cm², 0.1 W/cm² from day 4 to 8, and 30 J/cm², 0.3 W/cm² at day 8.

m-THPC concentrations were assessed in blood, tissue (tumour bronchus, pulmonary artery, lung, skin, muscle) and urine samples at vari-ous drug-light intervals by use of high performance liquid chromatography.[6]

RESULTS

Effect of m-THPC-PDT on tumour tissue

A dose of 0.075 mg *m*-THPC/kg and 10 J/cm² resulted in about 50% tumour necrosis (epithelial mesothelioma) due to tumour infarction, induced by tumour vessel wall necrosis and thrombosis. A typical watershed phenomenon was observed with a cuff of tumour cells of questionable viability around the thrombosed vessels and flank necrosis of tumour situated further away (Fig. 12.1).

A dose of 0.15 mg *m*-THPC/kg and 2 J/cm² resulted in a different pattern of tumour damage with ballooned tumour cells of questionable viability (biphasic mesothelioma).

A dose of 0.3 mg *m*-THPC/kg and 10 J/cm² delivered after 24 h resulted in a 10 mm deep complete tumour necrosis in the centre but preserved cells in the periphery of the treated areas, whereas no viable tumour cells were observed either in the centre or in the periphery when the same drug–light conditions were applied at a drug–light interval of 48 h. This holds true for both epithelial and biphasic mesothelioma.

m-THPC-PDT was effective in recurrent breast cancer with chest wall involvement, and tumour selectivity was enhanced if, for a drug dose of 0.3 mg *m*-THPC/kg, longer drug–light intervals were combined with an increased light dose (in terms of increased power density). At 4 d and 10 J/cm², 0.1 W/cm², tumour and flank skin necrosis occurred, whereas at 9 d and 30 J/cm², 0.3 W/cm², the tumour disappeared after a few days without damage of the overlying skin.

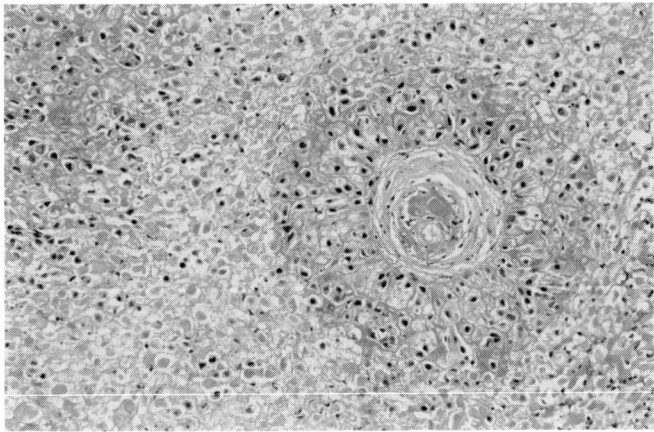

Fig. 12.1.   Tumour infarction, due to tumour vessel necrosis and thrombosis after *m*-THPC-PDT (0.075 mg *m*-THPC/kg 10 J/cm²). Histology 5 d after PDT. H & E × 100.

m-THPC pharmacokinetics

Plasma concentrations followed a first order kinetics with a half-time of 12 h. Nine days after administration, the compound was still detectable in the plasma. The results for two patients are shown in Table 12.1. No *m*-THPC or metabolites were measured in urine samples at any time point. There was a preferential uptake in tumour tissues, with tumour–skin ratio which varied from 3:1 to 14:1, and a tumour–bronchus ratio which varied from 4:1 to 6:1 at a drug–light interval of 48 h. The highest tumour–skin ratio was obtained for malignant histiocytoma (14:1). However, the drug concentration was a 100 times higher in plasma than in tissues after 48 h and tissue concentration measurements might have been biased by blood content or blood spilling.

Table 12.1.   Pharmacokinetics for *m*-THPC plasma concentrations in patients

Concentrations of drug – 48 h	(µg/g wet tissue)
Tumour	1.4
Bronchus	0.2
Pulmonary artery	0.3
Pulmonary vein	0.1
Skin	0.06
Muscle	0.2

Photobleaching

72 h after drug administration (0.3 mg/kg), *m*-THPC was measured in the tumour tissue (mesothelioma) before and just after light delivery (10 J/cm^2, 0.1 W/cm^2). A 75% decrease of *m*-THPC concentration in tumour tissue was observed after exposure to light, being 0.1467 µg/g tissue before PDT and 0.0379 µg/g after.

Skin photosensitivity

This occurred up to two and a half weeks after *m*-THPC administration was related to the *m*-THPC dose applied. In one patient skin necrosis occurred after exposure to bright light of an operating theatre lamp 24 h after administration of 0.3 mg *m*-THPC/kg.

Postoperative course

After intra-operative PDT following surgical tumour resection the postoperative course was marked by loss of appetite, fluid retention, hypoproteinemia and severe chest pain. One patient developed a colonic perforation on the left flexure 3 weeks after PDT although the diaphragm was debulked but left intact. The pattern of tissue damage was similar to that observed in tumour tissue after m-THPC-PDT. Temporary diversion colonostomy was performed and was reversed 2 months later.

One patient succumbed from aspiration-induced pneumonia of the contralateral lung after decortication and intra-operative m-THPC-PDT at the sixth postoperative day, giving a 30-d mortality of 13% after surgical tumour resection and intra-operative m-THPC-PDT of the chest involved. The autopsy of this patient revealed a 5 to 10 mm deep PDT necrosis of the remnant tumour (sarcomatous mesothelioma). Normal underlying structures such as the aorta, subclavian artery and brachial plexus, and the oesophagus were spared, even in the presence of a close relationship between tumour and normal tissues (Fig. 12.2).

Follow-up after intra-operative PDT following surgical tumour resection

No vascular or neural alterations were observed during follow-up, either on clinical grounds or on CT scans. One patient developed a small bronchopleural fistula after lobectomy (stapling technique) that did not require reoperation. The patients with plexus infiltration remained pain free without further neurological deterioration until death from tumour 4 months after the operation. All patients with mesothelioma developed distant metastases or contralateral disease during follow-up and six died 6 to 18

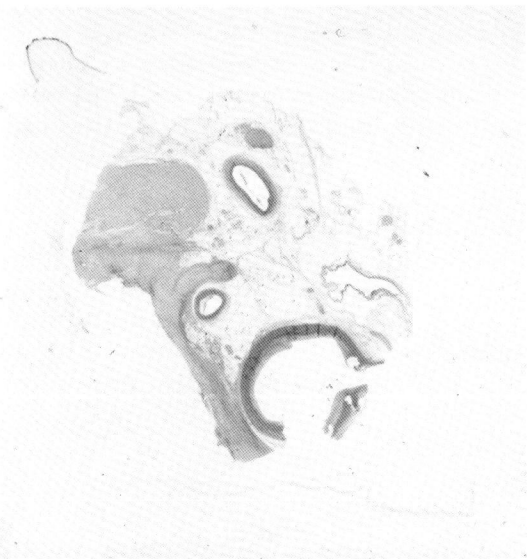

Fig. 12.2. Autopsy findings after intra-operative PDT of chest cavity. Cross-section through the pleural dome shows destroyed tumour and intact underlying subclavian artery.

months after the procedure. However, the areas treated 6 × PDT, first of all the diaphragm, remained free of gross tumour regrowth during follow up as judged on follow-up CT scans (Figure König). This holds also true for the patient with histiocytoma: no recurrence was found after 3 months at the diaphragm but recurrence developed in the untreated upper lobe (and pneumonectomy was performed).

DISCUSSION

Diffuse malignant pleural mesothelioma poses a difficult problem since there is no standard therapy for this usually fatal disease. All forms of treatment have failed to control tumour regrowth and improve survival. Because radiation and chemotherapy are relatively ineffective in mesothelioma[7-9], surgical resection has been considered the mainstay of treatment. However, the only prospective evaluation of surgery in malignant mesothelioma conducted by the Lung Cancer Study Group has failed to show any improvement of survival after surgical tumour resection compared to medical treatments or no treatment at all[10]. 20 selected patients underwent radical extrapleural pneumonectomy, but this did not result in better survival and 13 developed local recurrence during follow up. The information in the literature regarding the impact of a wide variety of treatments on survival is conflicting, but in all series, 5-year survival is exceptional for patients with malignant mesothelioma[11]. Therefore, new therapeutic approaches are warranted in this disease. Intra-operative PDT following surgical tumour resection might be an attractive new treatment concept, allowing for a selective clean up of the tumour bed after tumour removal with destruction of remnant disease while leaving underlying vital structures intact. Natural barriers against further tumour spread might be preserved, first of all the diaphragm. Moreover, PDT was effective in human malignant mesothelioma xenografts[12]. Since 1990, we have in a pilot study assessed PDT on selected patients suffering from malignant mesothelioma. Although the only sensitizer used in clinical trials at that time was haematoporphyrin derivatives (HpD), its efficacy and tumour selectivity was judged to be too low for intra-operative intrathoracic application[13]. Light must be delivered to large and geometrically complex surfaces bordered by vital structures which might be harmed by PDT, with detrimental sequelae.

In addition, treatment time and morbidity might be unduly increased if surgical tumour resection is followed by intra-operative PDT using HpD, given the high light dose required to induce tumour necrosis. Extrapleural pneumonectomy per se is a formidable procedure with an operative mortality ranging from 10%–20% in several series[14, 15]. To overcome the drawbacks of HpD, new sensitizers are currently being assessed under experimental and clinical conditions[16-18]. We have chosen *m*-THPC for our clinical pilot study since it is around 100 times more effective than HpD at inducing tumour necrosis, the effect being calculated on a depth of necrosis per mole of sensitizer basis. Moreover, it is activated at 650 nm, a wavelength with enhanced tissue penetration compared to 630 nm[19].

Our results indicated that the drug itself was well-tolerated and up to 0.3 mg/kg did not cause side effects other than skin photosensitivity. Skin photosensitivity was dose dependent and occurred up to two and a half weeks after drug administration. This time span is clearly smaller than that observed after HpD administration. However, photosensitivity after 0.3 mg m-THPC/kg may be severe and flank necrosis of skin was observed. Photosensitivity was considerably milder after administration of m-THPC (an m-THPC dose smaller than 0.3 mg/kg is required for further clinical application).

m-THPC concentration measurements revealed a first order kinetics for plasma concentrations with a half-life of 12 h. No m-THPC or metabolites were identified in urine samples, indicating that the drug is eliminated by hepatobiliary secretion. m-THPC tissue concentration measurements 48 h after drug administration indicated a tumour–skin ratio ranging from 3:1 to 14:1, and a tumour–bronchus ratio ranging from 4:1 to 6:1.

However, caution in the interpretation of these results is indicated since m-THPC concentrations were about 100 times higher in plasma than in tissues at that time point and tissue concentration measurements might have been biased by blood spilling of the tissue samples which were harvested for assessment. Our ongoing experimental results question the validity of m-THPC tissue concentration measurements as useful predictors of photosensitizing effects since they did not parallel the extent of tumour and normal tissue damage after m-THPC-PDT (in vivo on nude mice bearing human mesothelioma xenografts)[20].

m-THPC-PDT mediated deep tumour necrosis with relatively low light doses. A 10 mm deep tumour necrosis was obtained with only 10 J/cm^2 and 0.1 W/cm^2, which could not be attributed to thermal effects, given the low power density applied. This extent of necrosis was obtained for all histological types of mesothelioma (epithelial, biphasic and sarcomatous) and was clearly superior to that observed after HpD for this light dose. Tumour necrosis mediated seemed to be in first line the result of tumor infarction due to tumour vessel necrosis and thrombosis.

The autopsy findings of the patient dying 6 d after tumour resection and intra-operative PDT revealed that m-THPC-PDT is also effective if performed just after surgical tumour debulking, and the apparent absence of extensive muscle necrosis and of flank damage to bronchial, vascular and neural structures suggested some degree of tumour selectivity of m-THPC-PDT under clinical conditions. This is underscored by the postoperative course of the patient with plexus infiltration by mesothelioma. The pain disappeared only after PDT of the plexus involved but not after surgery alone, and no further neurological deficit was observed during follow-up.

The tissue selectivity of d-THPC-PDT might be in part attributed to the good photobleaching properties of *m*-THPC: a 75% decrease *m*-THPC concentration in tumour tissue was measured after application of 10 J/cm^2.

However, the postoperative course of our patients was marked by a significant additional morbidity, beyond that expected from surgery alone. Although the postoperative morbidity and mortality in this small series was comparable to that of other reports dealing with conventional surgery for this disease[10], major complications observed in our patients such as colonic perforation must be attributed to intra-operative *m*-THPC-PDT.

In order to enhance the therapeutic ratio of *m*-THPC-PDT, we assessed the extent of tumour and normal tissue damage on nude mice bearing human mesothelioma xenografts for various drug–light conditions and at drug–light intervals ranging from 4 h to 6 d. The results indicated that the therapeutic ratio can be considerably increased if, for a given drug dose, an increased light dose is delivered at longer drug–light intervals. Morbidity in our series was not decreased if light was delivered at 72 h instead of 48 h. However, PDT performed for recurrent breast cancer with chest-wall involvement revealed that the relation between drug–light conditions and therapeutic ration of *m*-THPC-PDT may behave similarly under clinical and experimental conditions, if longer drug–light intervals are used for clinical purposes. In this patient, 10 J/cm^2, 0.1 W/cm^2 delivered 4 d after administration of 0.3 mg *m*-THPC/kg resulted in flank necrosis of the tumour as well as of the overlying skin, but 30 J/cm^2, 0.3 W/cm^2 delivered 9 d after administration of the same drug dose resulted in tumour necrosis while the overlying skin was spared.

The follow-up of our patients underscores the necessity of offering a treatment modality with good local tumour control but minimal additional morbidity. Although repeated CT scans revealed no gross tumour regrowth of sites healed, and no alterations of vascular structures, all patients developed tumour spread to nodes, contralateral chest and to distant sites, and all but one patient died within a short period of time. It was believed that patients suffering from malignant mesothelioma succumb from relentless local progression of the disease[22]. Since better local tumour control is available, it becomes apparent that this tumour has a high metastatic potential and that only a multimodality approach might improve survival. Recurrent malignant histiocytoma is a rare tumour and only one patient was treated by PDT in this series. There was a preferential uptake of *m*-THPC in the tumour and tumour response was observed at sites treated by PDT as judged on follow-up CT scans, but no conclusion can be drawn, given the short follow up in this patient.

In summary, *m*-THPC is an effective second-generation sensitizer for photodynamic therapy. Intraoperative *m*-THPC-PDT is feasible under clinical conditions but is related to substantial additional morbidity if large surfaces are treated. A perfect tissue selectivity is mandatory for all effective new sensitizers which absorb strongly at longer wavelengths in order to prevent extensive damage to normal structures.

REFERENCES

1. Nambisan RN, Karakousis CP, Holyoke ED, Dougherty TJ 1988 Intraoperative photodynamic therapy for retroperitoneal sarcomas. Cancer 61: 1248–1252
2. Sindelar WF, DeLaney TF, Tochner Z, Thomas GF, Smith PD, Priauf WS, Gladstein E 1991 Technique of photodynamic therapy for disseminated intraperitoneal malignant neoplasms. Archives of Surgery 126: 318–324
3. Pass HI, Tochner Z, DeLaney T, Smith PD, Friauf WS, Glatstein E, Travis W 1990 Intraoperative photodynamic therapy for malignant mesothelioma. Letter to the editor. Annals of Thoracic Surgery 50: 687–688
4. Lofgren L, Larsson M, Thanning L, Hallgren S 1991 Transthoracic endoscopic photodynamic treatment of malignant mesothelioma. Lancet 337: 359
5. Berenbaum MC 1989 Comparison of hematoporphyrin derivatives and new photosensitizers. In: Photosensitizing compounds: their chemistry, biology and clinical use, Ciba Foundation Symposium 146. John Wiley and Sons, Chichester, 33–34
6. Wang Q, Ris MB, Altermatt HJ, Reynolds B, Stewart JCM, Bonnett R, Lim CK 1993 Determination of 5,10,15,20-Tetra m-hydroxyphenylchlorin in human plasma by high performance liquid chromatography. Biomedical Chromatography. 7: 45–47
7. Antmann KH, Li FP, Osteen R 1989 Mesothelioma. Cancer Updates 3: 1–16
8. Alberts AS, Falkson G, Goedhals L, Vorobiof DA, Van Der Merve CA 1988 Malignant pleural mesothelioma: a disease unaffected by current manoeuvres. Journal of Clinical Oncology 6: 527–34
9. Brady LW 1921 Mesothelioma – the role for radiation therapy. Seminars in Oncology 8: 329–34
10. Rusch VW, Piantadosi S, Holmes EC 1991 The role of extrapleural pneumonectomy in malignant pleural mesothelioma. A Lung Cancer Study Group trial. Journal of Thoracic and Cardiovascular Surgery 102: 1–9
11. Faber LP 1988 Surgical treatment of asbestos-related disease of the chest. Surgical Clinics of North America 68(3): 525–543
12. Feins RH, Hilf R, Ross H, Gibson SL 1990 Photodynamic therapy for human malignant mesothelioma in the nude mouse. Journal of Surgical Research 49: 311–314
13. Ris HB, Altermatt HJ, Inderbitzi R, Hess R, Nachbur B, Stewart JCM, Bonnett R, Berenbaum MC, Althaus U 1991 Photodynamic therapy with chlorins for diffuse malignant mesothelioma: initial clinical results. British Journal of Cancer 64: 1116–1120
14. Shemin RJ 1987 Surgical treatment of pleural mesothelioma. In: Antmann KH, Aisner J, (eds) Asbestos-related malignancy. Grune & Stratton, Orlando, pp 323–337
15. Butchart EG, 1989 Surgery of mesothelioma of the pleura. In: Roth JA, Ruckdeschel JC, Weisenburger TH, (eds) Thoracic oncology. WB Saunders Philadelphia, pp 556–583
16. Bonnett R, Berenbaum MC, 1989 Porphyrins as sensitizers. In: Photosensitizing compounds: their chemistry, biology and clinical use, Ciba Foundation Symposium 146. John Wiley and Sons, Chichester, 40–53
17. Van Lier JE, Spiles JD 1989 The chemistry, photophysics and photosensitizing properties of phthalocyanines. In: Photosensitizing compounds: their chemistry, biology and clinical use, Ciba Foundation Symposium 146. John Wiley and Sons, Chichester, pp 17–26
18. Pandey RK, Bellinier DA, Smith KM, Dougherty TJ 1991 Chlorin and porphyrin derivatives as potential photosenitizers in photodynamic therapy. Photochemistry and Photobiology 53: 65–72
19. Wilson BC, Patterson MS 1990 The determination of light influence distribution in photodynamic therapy. In: Kessel D (ed) Photodynamic therapy of neoplastic disease, vol 1. CRC Press, Boca Raton, pp 129–146
20. Ris HB, Altermatt HJ, Nachbur B, Stewart JCM, Wang Q, Lim CK, Bonnett R,

Ulthaus U 1993 Effect of drug–light interval on photodynamic therapy with meta-tetrahydroxyphenylchlorin in malignant mesothelioma. International Journal of Cancer 53: 141–461

21. Ris HB, Altermatt HJ, Nachbur B, Stewart JCM, Schaffner T, Wang Q, Lim CK, Bonnet R, Althaus U, 1993 Photodynamic therapy with *m*–tetrahydroxyphenylchlorin *in vivo*; optimization of the therapeutic index. International Journal of Cancer 55: 245–249

22. Nauta RJ, Osteen RT, Antmann KH, Koster JK, 1982 Clinical staging and the tendency of maligant pleural mesothelioma to remain localized. Annals of Thorac Surgery 34: 66–70

Index